SIX KEYS TO HEALING

Six Keys to Healing

and how to apply them

John Huggett

KINGSWAY PUBLICATIONS

EASTBOURNE

ISBN 0 86065 367 6

Unless otherwise indicated, biblical quotations are from
the New International Version, © New York International
Bible Society 1978.

Front cover design by Vic Mitchell

Many names in this book
have been changed in the interests
of confidentiality

Printed in Great Britain for
KINGSWAY PUBLICATIONS LTD
Lottbridge Drove, Eastbourne, E. Sussex BN23 6NT by
Cox & Wyman Ltd, Reading.
Typeset by CST, Eastbourne, E. Sussex.

To my darling wife, Chris,
without whose love, advice and patience
this book could never have been written,
and with heartfelt gratitude
to all those members of the Breath Fellowship
who have continually prayed for me
and encouraged me.

Contents

Foreword

How we all love a spiritual thriller! Christ walks into the room, new life pours into the dying man's body and he exclaims, 'I'm healed!' We pass the book around our circle of Christian friends, and what a lift it gives us. For a time anyway, then it's back to the normal ups and downs of Christian experience. Yes, the spiritual thriller has its place, and I know I have been helped many times by such books.

This book is different. It is thrilling but at a different level, very much like the different stories of people's conversions. Sometimes we are stirred by an exciting testimony of someone who has seen the light after a life of crime and wickedness. He has responded to the claims of Christ and his life has been transformed into a thing of beauty. We tell our friends about it, or refer to it in our sermons. We are thankful for such stories of the miracles of God's grace.

On the other hand, we have been greatly helped over the years by the quiet, consistent witness of fellow Christians in the local church with a less exciting testimony. They were brought up in Christian homes and committed their lives to Jesus at an early age, pressing on steadily from that point. John's book is akin to this second sort of testimony, solid and dependable.

At our church we have sought to encourage John and Chris in their work and this has given us many opportunities to meet them and see them in action. It was therefore a real pleasure for me to read this book; it was just like being with them because it is a living testimony of their healing ministry.

Six Keys to Healing is both winsome and encouraging. Many 'ordinary' Christians will identify with it; some will be 'drawn in' and others will be 'pulled along' in the realm of healing. The book is a basic manual on healing, but there is nothing cold and clinical about it—its pages are full of movement.

If you are looking for 'spiritual fireworks' this is not the book for you. But if you want something wholesome, dependable, strong and biblical, then read on—and remember the full title, '*Six Keys to Healing* and *How to Apply Them.*'

NORMAN BURROWS
Trinity Methodist Church, East Grinstead
Editor, Sound of Revival *magazine*

Take Out Your Keys

'Take out your keys.'

The voice in my mind was soft and gentle but as clear as a bell. Almost automatically I removed the ring of keys from my trouser pocket, for I sensed that God was speaking to me.

The congregation was singing a rousing hymn, and after that I was due to give the final address of our 1982 healing mission to Doncaster. At each of the six meetings I'd preached about a different key to healing, but it was only now as I glanced at the ring that I discovered that there were six keys on it. I drew the attention of the congregation to this as I began to preach.

After the service I noticed something more: a definite correlation between each key on the ring and each key I'd preached about.

Take my front-door key to start with. It was one of those small Yale keys that have to be firmly pressed into the lock before turning. This reminded me of the first key to be applied in healing—the front-door key of *faith*. Without faith in Christ prayer for healing is ineffective, yet through faith gigantic mountains of sickness can be removed.

My back-door key was much bulkier, one of those heavy, long-barrelled ones that tended to weigh down the others in my pocket. When I began to ask myself what was behind the healing ministry I knew it was the *guidance* of the Holy Spirit. Only as I'm walking in the Lord's will can I expect to see his power effective in healing.

A third and much smaller key on my ring fitted the fuel tank in our car. The lock on that tank was generally hidden from view as a shutter could be closed over it to provide additional protection. This key reminded me of the vital key of *love*. Not long beforehand, a Pentecostal pastor had made an interesting remark when he'd invited me to speak to his church. 'I've been here for over twenty years,' he'd said, 'and we've had ministry for healing at our services regularly. But I cannot say we've had much success in this area when you consider how long we've been doing it. Could we be missing something?'

'I'm not sure,' I'd replied. But the pastor's observation had tied in with something the Lord was impressing on me in a fresh way: Christians are sometimes quick to blame lack of success on lack of faith, but faith is not the only key required. It's often love which breaks through to the hidden inner realms of people's minds and memories that also need healing. Perhaps it was for this reason that when I spoke to the pastor's church my message was about love . . . .

Then I came to the fourth key on my ring, a funny-looking wedge-shaped one that fitted the door of our garage. I recalled how tools are often kept in the garage and how my wife Chris and I had discovered that we could not do our particular healing ministry without some vital tools—the *gifts* of the Holy Spirit.

Next there was the large black ignition key to our car. This spoke to me of God's *power*—the key to spiritual ignition. We'd experienced some services where faith and love were in evidence but the power of the Spirit was not released through praise, gifts or ministry.

The remaining key on my ring, a flat squarish one, fitted every door of the car, including the boot-lid and the cubby-hole. Without this key we were unable to get into our vehicle, let alone move forward in it. I concluded that a willingness to *change* was the key to Christian progress, and is often necessary for complete wholeness.

Gathering up the bunch of keys I slipped them back into my pocket, wondering how I could make use of what the Lord had pointed out to me.

My first opportunity came the same year. The six keys to healing formed the themes of our first six cassettes. The messages on these are the basis of this book. Meanwhile our ministry was developing in other ways too. You can read the full story of how it was born out of pain and suffering and how it began to develop in *It Hurts to Heal* (Kingsway Publications 1984).

Many people wanted to know more than the basic insights about the keys shared in these addresses. 'We've learned a lot about the what and the why,' they remarked, 'but we want to know more about the how and the when.'

So we began a series of training days at East Grinstead on applying the keys to healing. These days were attended by Christians from near and far, and were later repeated in other districts. We discussed many practical questions like 'How should we pray for the sick?', 'Should we expect instant results?', 'When should I lay hands on someone?' and 'How can I share the gifts of the Spirit with a sick person?' The cream of what we studied during those days is reproduced in this book.

We are living in exciting times because there's a great resurgence of interest in supernatural healing all over the world. Chris and I have been privileged to see and hear of hundreds of people healed through our prayers, but our great desire is to help more believers share the healing of

Jesus with those in need.

Especially for the benefit of readers new to Christian healing, the first two chapters of this book deal with its foundations. The remaining chapters explore in depth the six keys to healing and how to apply them.

My prayer is that you will discover much as you read these pages with Jesus Christ who is 'the same yesterday and today and for ever' (Heb 13:8) and who is therefore able to meet every need.

John Huggett

Six Keys to Healing

There are six different keys
    That we can use in healing.
The Lord who gave us these
    Is to his church appealing.
Faith is the front-door key,
    And, if we will believe it,
Though health we cannot see,
    Through Jesus we'll receive it.

Another key we need
    For Jesus to restore us:
It is to let him lead,
    For he would go before us.
To unlock mind and soul
    And heal deep pains and tension,
His key that makes us whole
    Is love which breathes compassion.

As word and touch we share,
    His gifts are here to guide us.
The tools are always there,
    And Jesus stands beside us.
There is release of power
    And spiritual ignition:
So healing flows that hour,
    Deliverance and salvation.

The final key we use:
    We're willing and committed
To do what Christ shall choose,
    For holiness be fitted.
We use your mighty name,
    Lord Jesus, you're our healer,
And you we shall proclaim
    For ever and for ever.

FOUNDATIONS OF CHRISTIAN HEALING

I

The Longest Arms in the World

The cleverest criminals, thinking they've escaped justice by fleeing to other countries, have sometimes been startled by the arrival of the police. The 'long arm of the law' has reached across the miles and grasped hold of them.

God's arms are ten thousand times longer and stronger, but they are also arms of love and gentleness.

'All day long I have stretched out My hands to people unyielding and disobedient' (Rom 10:21 Amplified Version).

'How often I have longed to gather your children together, as a hen gathers her chicks under her wings' (Mt 23:37).

'He gathers the lambs in his arms and carries them close to his heart; he gently leads those that have young' (Is 40:11).

The world is torn apart by suffering, and countless sick people have not been healed, even after much prayer. So we could easily conclude that God doesn't care about them, until we recall the longings of Jesus:

'When Jesus landed and saw a large crowd, he had

compassion on them and healed their sick' (Mt 14:14).

'Filled with compassion, Jesus reached out his hand and touched the man. "I am willing," he said. "Be clean!" Immediately the leprosy left him and he was cured' (Mk 1:41–42).

God longs to heal us—but how do we know he wants to?

HE MADE US

Christians believe that God gave us life and gave our parents power to bring us into the world.

A housewife is peeling potatoes. Her knife slips and she accidentally cuts herself. New cells form and the wound heals over, for the human body is the most wonderful of all machines and has a built-in repair system. This is just one evidence that when God formed us he planned and expected healing for us.

HE LOVES US

My wife once woke up in the middle of the night with a violent pain. As it showed no sign of subsiding I telephoned the doctor, automatically assuming that he'd be willing to help. It never occurred to me that he'd say, 'No, I don't want your wife to be well.' I expected the doctor to do all he could, and he did.

Yet there's a widespread idea that God is less concerned than doctors. Some Christians even think they have to get him into a good mood before he'll be willing to heal them. One lady with this belief shared it with her psychiatrist and his understandable response was, 'Your God is too terrible for words!'

But God is the exact opposite. We see what he's really like by looking at Jesus. He healed people not primarily to prove he was God but because he *is* God. He just couldn't help ministering to them. His heart went out to them whatever their needs. He summarized what he came to do when he read Isaiah's words in the synagogue: 'The Spirit of the Lord is on me, because he has anointed me to preach good news to the poor. He has sent me to proclaim freedom for the prisoners and recovery of sight for the blind, to release the oppressed, to proclaim the year of the Lord's favour' (Lk 4:18–19; cf. Is 61:1–2).

We learn about God's concern, too, from the followers of Jesus. Peter describes the Lord as 'not wanting anyone to perish, but everyone to come to repentance' (2 Pt 3:9). So when people remain unsaved it's not God's fault—they need to repent. Similarly, God doesn't want anyone to be sick but everyone to be made whole. Ideally we'd all die of old age not disease. So when people remain unhealed we have no right to blame God.

When I visited Dora, a lady with arthritis, she remarked, 'I suppose this trouble is the cross I have to bear.'

'Did you voluntarily decide to have arthritis, then?' I asked her.

'Oh no!' she replied.

'Well, the cross Christians are called to carry is one they pick up voluntarily,' I explained. 'We can expect to bear suffering but sickness and disease are part of the evil in the world, things Jesus died to save us from. The Lord doesn't want you to put up with your arthritis. He loves you far too much for that.'

Dora looked into my eyes and asked abruptly, 'You don't think it's a punishment, then? Something sent to try me?'

I replied by referring to my grown-up sons, Stephen and Paul.

'When they were younger,' I recalled, 'they misbehaved at times. I can't say I've been a very good father, but when I disciplined them I don't ever remember saying, "This is the way I'll punish you: I'm going to make you sick." Now I'm certain that God's a much better father than I am, and I'm equally sure that he loves you enough to want you well and healthy.'

HE HAS PROMISED TO HEAL US

The Bible is full of God's promises to heal (see appendix). There are 127 references to health and healing, and there was no commission given to Jesus' first disciples that did not include healing.

James' advice is also the word of God to Christian people: 'Is any one among you sick? He should call in the church elders . . . And they should pray over him, anointing him with oil in the Lord's name. And the prayer [that is] of faith will save him that is sick, and the Lord will restore him; and if he has committed sins, he will be forgiven' (Jas 5: 14–15 Amplified Version).

'What about Paul's thorn in the flesh?' I'm sometimes asked. 'Since God didn't take it away after Paul had prayed three times (2 Cor 12:7–9), doesn't that show that God may sometimes not wish to heal the sick?' Although the idea is popular that Paul's thorn was a sickness, this is by no means certain. It's called 'a messenger of Satan', and on every other occasion that the Greek word for 'messenger' is used it refers to a person, or an angel. So Paul's thorn may well have been a person who constantly annoyed him. Today we might call such a person not a thorn in the flesh but a pain in the neck.

But even if it was a sickness, it was the exception rather than the rule. Paul didn't teach that God's normal plan for the world included disease. Sickness clearly resulted from sin and man's fall. If we believe otherwise, why do we go to the doctor? Why don't we throw away our tablets and thank God for our ill health?

We can claim, then, God's promises to heal from Scripture.

Sometimes sick people also receive promises of healing through prophecy, which should accord with God's written word. Fay, a lady in the north of England, suffered with rheumatoid arthritis. She was given a promise that she'd be completely healed, but there was no immediate outward sign of this. Fay wisely did not stop receiving ministry, and one day three years later she suddenly found that the Lord had healed her.

HE HAS DEMONSTRATED HIS HEALING POWER

'God anointed Jesus of Nazareth with the Holy Spirit and power, and . . . he went around . . . healing all who were under the power of the devil' (Acts 10:38).

Approximately two thirds of Jesus' ministry was taken up with healing the sick. And though he didn't rush through the streets and lanes of the Holy Land in search of sick people, every single one that bothered to come to him he healed. He didn't say to one person, 'I willingly restore you,' and to the person who came next, 'Sorry, I don't wish to make you better.'

When Jesus died on the cross it wasn't only to save us from sin, but that by his stripes we might be healed (Is 53:5). That is why Matthew, referring to the prophecy about God's suffering servant, writes, 'He . . . restored to health all who were sick; and thus he fulfilled what was spoken by the prophet Isaiah, He himself took . . . our weaknesses and infirmities and bore away our diseases' (Mt 8:16–17 Amplified Version).

Picture a crippled woman in great pain entering your local church and longing to be cured. Her doctor would hope for her recovery. You and the congregation presumably would not want constant pain and disease for her. And surely the Lord would be the most willing of all to see her made whole. If Jesus was standing in that church building and that woman asked him to heal her there's no doubt that he would. But Jesus is in the church, for he lives in his people by his Spirit and is able through them to bring healing.

It's true that while the Lord doesn't normally send sickness he allows it, just as he allowed Satan to cover Job's body with painful sores (Job 2:7).

All over the world God is triumphing over sickness and disease. More people are becoming Christians and more people are being healed through prayer than at any other period in history. There's abundant evidence that God wants to heal.

How do we see God's healing?

THROUGH MEDICINE

Jesus said, 'It is not the healthy who need a doctor, but the sick' (Mt 9:12). When we see doctors, nurses and psychiatrists bringing about healing we're observing God at work. Many of them are unaware that they are his healing agents.

This is important to grasp because some Christians, having discovered healing through prayer, are ignoring the God-given gift of medicine. Like all good gifts it can be abused, but it's still the way through which God brings healing to the majority.

Doctor Luke, who probably wrote the Acts of the Apostles, is zealous about 'Christian healing'. But he also uses many medical terms, and seems to have combined his medical experience with his spiritual gifts.

The Lord is wonderfully healing many thousands of sick folk today through supernatural gifts, but he uses what medical men and women have discovered too. Some of these discoveries are controversial, but so are some discoveries that Christians have made.

One evening at a healing service, during the laying-on-of-hands, a woman asked me to pray for a new kidney for her sister. It so happened that I'd recently watched a television programme about kidney donors. Apparently there were many of these in the country, but because of a lack of communication the kidneys were not always made available on time. So I prayed that a new kidney would become available for this woman's sister.

The next day the woman came up to my wife Chris and said indignantly, 'When I asked your husband to pray for a new kidney for my sister I didn't mean a transplant—that's second-hand—I meant a new one. God can do it.'

'Of course he can,' Chris agreed. 'But he doesn't only use supernatural methods to answer our prayers. In fact much of the time he uses natural means. The important thing is that we don't limit God to any one way of working.'

But the woman remained unconvinced.

My own experience, however, backs up what Chris said. I once suffered an acute mental breakdown characterized by exaggerated fears and anxieties. My complete healing took over eighteen months and many things contributed to it: medical and psychiatric help, drugs and the process of time, prayer and ministry, the help and encouragement of my wife and friends and, in the latter stages, the fact that I did much to help myself.

Christians, however, will often wish to consult the Lord before sending for the doctor. We also need much guidance about the vast range of 'alternative therapies' that are available today. Some of these, like osteopathy, are frequently the Lord's provision. Others, like spiritist healing, are counterfeits of true, divine healing.

Many other therapies need to be checked out against God's word before we make use of them. Meditation, for example, can be beneficial if Christian but dangerous if transcendental. We even need to check the credentials of Christian healers, some of whom are not working from Scripture or with the churches. While a measure of healing can be obtained through various means, complete wholeness will include getting right with God through repentance and faith in the Lord Jesus Christ.

I look forward to seeing more co-operation between

medical authorities and Christian ministers of healing.

Meanwhile, prayer can often aid the doctors. When I was Curate at Buckhurst Hill in Essex we prayed for eleven-weeks-old Rebecca who was seriously ill with a circulatory problem. After a crucial four-hour heart operation Rebecca was restored to her parents. The local press described this as a 'miracle cure', but Peter the Rector explained to them, 'We asked God to guide the hand of the surgeon. I believe we have perhaps created the right spiritual environment for the child to recover in.'

After the leper was cleansed Jesus said, 'Go, show yourself to the priest' (Mt 8:4). The priest would be able to confirm the cure.

Today the medical training and experience of doctors enable them to perform a similar function. After we'd ministered to a lady with stomach cancer, X-rays showed that the cancer had stopped in its tracks and then gradually diminished. Many doctors have been surprised at the evidence of their own eyes in confirming what Christians had prayed for.

THROUGH MINISTRY

Paul writes about gifts of healing given to believers on particular occasions to share with those in need (1 Cor 12:9). Some Christians, such as Chris and myself, exercise ministries of healing which means that we're frequently involved with sick people. But every Christian can share in some way in healing, and I'm thrilled that in many churches this is becoming a normal part of what is happening. (I will be discussing the distinction between gifts and ministry in a later chapter.)

This ministry is usually to the whole person—body, soul and spirit—and it may be for healing of relationships too. When ministering forgiveness of sin we often call the end product salvation. Restoration of body, mind and emotions to a healthy condition we call healing. Setting free from bondages and satanic influences we refer to as deliverance. But in the New Testament the same Greek word is often used for all three, and the terms are interchangeable. God doesn't see us as bits and pieces but as whole persons, so he doesn't do things by halves.

Christians minister healing in Jesus' name through speech. This may involve spoken prayer. They are sometimes given words of knowledge through which they are shown by the Lord what the need is or how he will deal with it (1 Cor 12:8). And as we speak out the authoritative word of God it frequently brings healing.

Chris was once invited to a women's meeting to speak about what Jesus is doing today. At the close Elsie, the elderly lady leading the meeting, asked Chris to pray for her. 'It's my legs,' she said wearily. 'I've had them in bandages for fifteen years now. It's an incurable skin disease. They weep all the time.'

My wife knelt on the floor and laid her hands on Elsie's legs to pray. Immediately Chris closed her eyes she discerned that the disease was caused by an evil spirit, so before praying for healing she rebuked the condition in Jesus' name.

I believe it was because Chris prayed in this way that within a few days Elsie was healed completely. 'Look,' she said excitedly, 'my legs! I can actually see my legs! I'm wearing stockings for the first time in fifteen years!'

It was so encouraging to observe Elsie's joy, and Chris felt she herself was the one who'd been blessed.

Many Christians have discovered that the ministry of touch frequently adds to the effectiveness of spoken prayer and the spoken word. Jesus didn't just speak to people, he often stretched out his hand and touched them. Sometimes it was on the affected part of the body, such as the blind man's eyes (Jn 9:6).

Chris and I lay hands on people in healing services, but it also seems natural to touch them whenever they need prayer, and so let the Lord's power flow through our hands to meet their needs.

Sometimes we minister soaking prayer. We keep our hands on the affected part of a person's body for a lengthy period and allow the healing energy to 'soak in' while we pray, worship in song or talk informally.

The laying-on-of-hands gives specific opportunities to receive direct ministry, and if it's rightly received the needy person is always blessed in some way. This also applies when someone stands proxy for an absent sick person, just as the centurion came to Jesus for his slave who was ill at home (Mt 8:5–13).

Sometimes the spoken word would be unintelligible to the needy person. This was so in the case of a mentally-retarded boy brought to me during a healing service. Although he could not follow my words he could feel my touch, and that, I believe, was the touch of Jesus. Twelve months later I met the boy's parents at another service and they told me how their son had so improved that he was taking his GCEs.

It seems pointless to preach and teach about healing without giving those present an opportunity to experience the touch of Jesus for themselves. While they may do this right where they are, many have testified to the additional blessings received through coming forward for the laying-on-of-hands. It's a public witness that they mean business with God and it's a wonderful witness that he's still full of compassion and longing to heal.

God's arms are still the longest in the world.

Suggested readings: Jeremiah 30:10–17 and James 5:13–20.

2

A Present from Doctor Jesus

Doctors are in the habit of handing out prescriptions, and some people consider visits to the surgery a waste of time unless they come away clutching those little slips of paper.

Jesus had no written prescription to offer, but he didn't dispense the gift of healing casually. It was so precious to him that he arranged for it to be made available after his ascension, and the gift has been passed on down the centuries.

God has never stopped healing—but how has the church reacted?

THE EARLY PERIOD

When Jesus first sent out his twelve apostles 'they went out and preached that people should repent. They drove out many demons and anointed many sick people with oil and healed them' (Mk 6:12–13). But the task of healing wasn't confined to the twelve. The seventy (or seventy-two) 'laymen' were also commanded to do it (Lk 10:9).

The chief opponents of this ministry were the Jewish religious leaders. Today, too, the chief critics of the Christian healing ministry are not doctors or unbelievers but church leaders. That's why some churches are apathetic about it.

A vicar was taken ill and went into hospital. His parochial church council was meeting that week but instead of praying for his healing they sent him a message: 'We wish you a speedy recovery by eleven votes to ten.'

Perhaps because Jesus was aware that not all would receive the message of healing, he didn't confine his commission before his ascension to the eleven either. It was to them that he said, 'Go into all the world and preach the good news to all creation' (Mk 16:15). But he added, 'These signs will accompany those who believe . . . they will place their hands on sick people, and they will get well' (Mk 16:17–18).

All believers have been commissioned to share the gift; all who put their faith in Christ for salvation and trust him to heal. Leaders have an important part to play, but the gift belongs to the whole body of Christ.

Jesus ministered in a variety of ways: in public or in private, by touch or by word. And there was a variety of healing methods used by the early Christians too.

However, nearly all prayers for healing in the New Testament share a common feature—they are not request prayers like 'Lord, please make Michael's legs better', but command prayers like 'In the name of Jesus Christ of Nazareth, walk' (Acts 3:6). Today we tend to use request prayers, but we may need more command ones if we're to see a measure of healing similar to the early church.

In the New Testament sick people are nearly always instantly healed. Every so often in our own ministry a person that we pray for is cured instantaneously. At one healing service we laid hands on a deaf man and his hearing was immediately restored. After the service there was a sandwich tea. People were used to shouting at the man and they did this during the tea, but he said, 'It's all right,

I can hear now.'

Most healings today, however, are gradual. Why then were there so many instant healings in the early church?

One reason is that people came for ministry without the intellectual prejudices of the modern Western world. Another is that today's pressures make much more healing of the emotions necessary, and this by nature is usually gradual.

God has his own spiritual laws within which he works. Just as the surgeon must have all the correct facilities present before he can perform his operation, so only if all the circumstances are suitable will the Lord effect complete healing immediately. A lack of one of the keys discussed in this book may delay healing.

One secret of the effectiveness of the early church that many Christians are rediscovering today is a release of power in the Holy Spirit. Jesus healed only after his anointing by the Spirit at his baptism. The first Christians also had a similar experience. While Jesus was on earth in body they drew their power to heal from his presence, but once he left them they had to wait for the Spirit to descend before going out again to preach and heal.

One member of the infant church who worked signs and wonders was Stephen (Acts 6:8). He was only a deacon, but he was 'full of faith and of the Holy Spirit' (Acts 6:5).

Another was Philip, the evangelist. Like Jesus he often healed people in the context of preaching and teaching. The signs and wonders confirmed the truth of the message proclaimed, but they were also a means of attracting people to hear the word: 'When the crowds heard Philip and saw the miraculous signs he did, they all paid close attention to what he said. With shrieks, evil spirits came out of many, and many paralytics and cripples were healed' (Acts 8:6–7).

Christian healing is still a marvellous point of contact for evangelism. At a church service in East Grinstead a young couple brought their ten-month-old baby to be prayed for. 'Rebecca has a discharge from her ears,' they explained. 'It's been going on for some time and the doctors say if it doesn't clear up soon they'll have to operate.'

Everyone was quiet, uniting in prayer as we laid hands on the child and prayed. In a few days the discharge had cleared up and the operation was unnecessary. The little girl was so obviously blessed that a neighbour noticed and Rebecca's parents were able to lead this woman to accept Jesus as her own Saviour.

Christian healing continued to flourish for about 300 years after Jesus ascended. Irenaeus, a bishop in the second century, wrote, 'None who believe in Christ and call on his name remain unhealed.' Augustine writing in the fourth century declared, 'We see there are miracles at this day wrought by God.'

Early in the fourth century Constantine became the Holy Roman Emperor and was eventually baptized as a Christian. Christianity became the official religion of the empire and it became 'the thing to do' to go to church. Consequently thousands who had no genuine faith began calling themselves Christians, thus fewer people had the simple faith required to expect healing.

At the same time medicine, which had tended to be comparatively primitive, was making tremendous strides forward and many people were in effect thinking 'Now we have medicine we can't expect miracles any more.' The consequence was that Christian healing fell into disrepute.

THE CENTURIES BETWEEN

The ministry of Christian healing never died out completely and there are countless instances of individual saints working miracles. But for over 1,500 years the prevailing attitude to sickness in the church was to be a fatalistic one.

When Christians marched against Mohammedans in the Crusades, for example, their beliefs about disease and death were not very different from those of their enemies who would say resignedly, 'It is the will of Allah.' Medicines and herbs would be used to alleviate suffering, but prayer for God to spare the sick in mercy would be qualified by phrases like 'if it is your will'.

This is a phrase which Chris and I never use in prayer for healing because it normally is God's will to heal. By adding this phrase we are adding doubt to our requests, and that does nothing to encourage the person we're ministering to. Sometimes we do need to discover God's will about *how* he will heal. Should someone have an operation? Or should he trust the Lord to restore him without it?

When a Christian is very old it may be God's will to heal him by taking him to be with himself. However, we once assumed God would do this when we laid hands on one old man and instead he was given several more years of life and health! There are many mysteries in healing and much that we still have to learn, but when people do die after being prayed for they often do so quickly and painlessly.

All this is a far cry from what happened in the church during the Middle Ages and even after the Reformation. Predominantly, sickness was viewed as God's judgement on people. Suffering was hailed as a virtue and to bear sickness stoically was therefore praised. While today we admire how some people cope with their sickness, or turn their disabilities to good advantage, we pray too for their complete healing.

Throughout the centuries, then, though Christians played leading parts in the foundation of hospitals and orphanages, they did comparatively little to encourage a healing ministry through positive prayer.

Yet there were some voices in the darkness. Martin

Luther in the sixteenth century said, 'It still does happen that by calling on his name [Christ] the sick have been healed.' Count Zinzendorf in the eighteenth century declared, 'I testify that apostolic powers are manifested . . . we have undeniable proof of the healing of incurable maladies by prayer.' And William Booth in the nineteenth century wrote, 'The recent remarkable signs and wonders [of healing] wrought among us demand our consideration. I believe in the necessity of these gifts.' Whenever there has been a genuine spiritual revival there has also been a resurgence of this ministry. John Wesley recorded 200 different cases of divine healing in his famous journal. The 'healing light' has never been extinguished.

It's only since the end of the nineteenth century, however, that there's been a real restoration of the healing ministry, and this began with the Pentecostal movement.

By this time some scholars had put forward neatly 'tied-up' explanations of why miracles didn't usually happen any more. They were written off either as part of the 'mythology' of the New Testament or they were said to have ceased with the closure of the apostolic age.

The Pentecostals refused to accept either explanation. Encouraged by their rediscovery of other gifts of the Holy Spirit, like prophecy and tongues, they were soon manifesting gifts of healing as well. But the orthodox churches in general didn't like their message or methods, so they were forced out of the 'mainline' churches in spite of their influence upon the Welsh Revival and of wonderful miracles performed through men of God like Smith Wigglesworth, the Bradford plumber.

Wigglesworth, who was given tremendous gifts of faith, would frequently lay hands on the sick and countless people were healed through him. But his work was often opposed by religious leaders, as once happened in Sweden where he was told he could only speak at a rally if he didn't lay hands on anyone. Undeterred, he encouraged the sick to lay their own hands on the affected parts of their bodies while he prayed. Hundreds were healed and converted as a result.

THE PRESENT DAY

Meanwhile, some Anglicans were recognizing the value of the gift. James Moore Hickson, encouraged by some bishops, exercised a worldwide healing ministry. Healing homes were established like Dorothy Kerin's at Burswood and George Bennett's at Crowhurst. Healing guilds such as the Order of St Luke were set up. Healing evangelists appeared on the scene, and healing missions like the London Healing Mission sprang up. But, in spite of all these, many people tended to equate non-medical healing with spiritism, Christian science, or even white witchcraft. Healing in the churches was generally a Cinderella.

It's been the charismatic renewal, beginning in this country in the 1960s, that has brought to thousands a new expectation that God will work visibly. So many have had a new experience of the Holy Spirit's power and gifts that every major denomination has been affected, including the Roman Catholics. The 1970s have seen the spread of charismatic communities and the rise of house churches, both involved with healing, and the 1980s have brought official recognition of the healing ministry from high-ranking church leaders.

During the last fifty years all the great biblical miracles have been paralleled in spiritual revivals.

One of the circumstances that sparked off the Indonesian revival was when a young Christian, afflicted with blindness and lameness through tampering with the occult, confessed his sins and testified in church. It was only a matter of hours afterwards that over fifty people became Christians. The ensuing period saw believers turning water into wine for communion, walking across water to preach the gospel to natives, and even raising the dead.

In one part of Canada homes were reunited in the Lord, family relationships were healed and businesses were cleansed from corruption.

In the Solomon Islands a man was ministered to who had been crippled for eight years with his knees bent up under his chin. His legs began to shake and as they did they became loose and straightened. Then a rushing mighty wind swept through the local community causing many to cry out with conviction of sin. Similar instances have occurred in Korea, parts of Africa and South America.

Elsie Salmon, a famous healing evangelist in South Africa, once declared, 'A spiritual revival could not come in a better way than through the healing of body, mind, soul and spirit. This is the greatest challenge the church has received in this generation—divine healing.'

Today healing evangelists like Oral Roberts of America and Trevor Dearing of England have an important part to play. But as the healing ministry receives more recognition as a normal part of the church's work, it's becoming more popular for Christians to minister to one another too.

In many parts of the UK you'll have no difficulty in finding at least one church where there's a regular healing service, laying-on-of-hands at communion, or a prayer group for the sick. I rejoice that the present from Doctor Jesus is at last being taken seriously again and being made available through his body, the church.

There are two subtle dangers, however. Firstly, if the pendulum swings the other way and healing becomes 'too respectable', it will just be another ceremony to be 'got through', 'having a form of godliness but denying its power' (2 Tim 3:5).

Secondly, the gift could become limited to being shared by ordained ministers alone, or quietly relegated to an off-peak hour at the communion rail. While the Lord has used some pastors to heal like this, we need to take the risk (with all its problems) of making the gift available to the whole body and as a major part of the church's programme. Then not only will God's people find their own needs met, but outsiders will discover that Jesus is relevant to their situations too.

How are Christians responding?

RED-LIGHT BELIEVERS AND THEIR PROBLEMS

Some Christians remain at a stand-still with regard to the healing ministry because they are ignorant or unconcerned. Others are happy to receive healing but content to leave sharing it to ministers and specialists, often feeling inadequate for the task themselves. Those who have the compassion of Jesus but are still waiting at the red light frequently voice two doubts.

Firstly, they do not believe that God can use them to bring healing to others. A lady whose eyesight remarkably improved after Chris and I had ministered to her, expressed her gratitude to us for being God's channels but seemed astonished to learn that God could use her to bring healing to others. Yet Jesus said, 'Everything is possible for him who believes' (Mk 9:23).

Can anyone learn to paint? Probably not to the extent of a master artist, but nearly everyone can do some painting and develop the ability if they wish. It's the same with healing. Obviously the Christian will grow more confident as he gains experience in using the gift, but the same Jesus who has brought healing to millions indwells him by the same Holy Spirit.

Secondly, they say that the healing ministry isn't practical. 'Our church isn't interested,' they remark.

The local church is, in fact, the best place for the healing ministry. But until every church practises it there's a need for interdenominational fellowships like ours where Christians can minister to one another across denominational barriers.

GREEN-LIGHT BELIEVERS AND THEIR PROGRESS

While some Christians wait at an amber light for a thunderbolt from heaven, many realize that God's green light is beckoning them to get moving now. And they are finding that as they step out so they are given all that they need for each task.

Healing is a costly business in terms of time, patience and everything. But for those who are willing to learn—from the Lord, from the Scriptures, from Christian teachers and from their own mistakes—it's exciting and fulfilling.

A frequent comment at some of our training days has been, 'I never realized there was so much to it as this.' Other folk have returned with joy, like the disciples of old, reporting on what God has done through them as a result of their stepping out in faith (Lk 10:17).

I've learned a lot personally by watching other ministers of healing at work, and above all by reading the Gospels and seeing the Great Physician himself at work. If you can get to Christian healing services you'll find they differ, but you'll probably be encouraged by what you see and hear and so find confidence to minister yourself.

But there's no substitute for actually doing it as the Holy Spirit leads you. As Francis of Assisi said, 'It is in giving that we receive.'

That's what this book is all about. We Christians have held the precious gift of healing in our hands for too long. It's time that we shared it more, and we need to learn how and when. It's time we looked more closely at the keys to healing and how to apply them.

Suggested readings: Mark 16:14–20 and Acts 8:4–8.

Key 1

FAITH: THE FRONT DOOR KEY TO LIVING

3

'Somebody Touched My Clothes!'

On at least two occasions Chris and I have been locked out of our house because we've forgotten to take a front-door key and there's been no one to let us in. In each case it was some time before we gained entry.

Similarly, without the front-door key of faith Christians can make no headway in healing. We need to carry it with us all the time, for there can be no ministry of faith without a life of faith.

When is faith essential?

Faith is always necessary for complete wholeness—for all a person's needs to be met (Acts 16:31).

SIMPLE FAITH FOR PERSONAL SALVATION

Some people have suffered physically, mentally or emotionally for many years. We reassure them with the reminder that Jesus heals long-term complaints, but we stress that the long-term complaint we all need healing from is sin. We mustn't dodge the sin problem. So we can encourage someone to receive healing of his relationship with God, but he must personally repent and put his faith in Christ for this. At this stage the important thing is not how much faith he has but that he definitely commits himself to the Lord.

When we are counselling we often need to discover where a person stands spiritually. Does he need to be converted? To find assurance? To return to God after backsliding? To recommit his life? Sometimes Christians find the answer as the Lord puts words or pictures into their minds. But frequently it comes as we ask questions like 'Have you a faith?' or 'Have you received ministry before?' Once we have diagnosed the need we can minister accordingly.

A helpful way of 'clinching' a conversion is encouraging an enquirer to say a prayer of commitment after you phrase by phrase. This ideally should include thanks to the Lord that he has come into the person's life. Yet this is just the beginning of a costly growth, and the spiritual babe will need care, food, fellowship and encouragement.

Some Christians are more gifted than others at leading people to accept salvation, and in the work of evangelism often 'one sows and another reaps' (Jn 4:37). But in one sense every Christian should be a reaper, just as every available farmhand is called in to help at harvest time. The church has plenty of sowers but not enough reapers, so more of us need to step out in faith.

SEED-FAITH FOR PHYSICAL RESTORATION

The Lord's not only looking for a harvest of converts but a harvest of healing. This will mean planting the seed of faith for healing in people's hearts and giving it time to grow as they respond to our ministry. Then, since 'a man reaps what he sows' (Gal 6:7), if we've sown the healing of Jesus we'll reap healthy Jesus people.

However, it's sometimes lack of faith in the Lord which is the blockage restricting or delaying healing. At Nazareth Jesus was faced with such a barrier of unbelief that even he 'could not do any miracles there' (Mk 6:5). When the person in need and the Christian ministering to him both exercise faith, that aids healing. When one or other of them fails to exercise faith, that can obstruct healing.

At a Bristol meeting I ministered to two women in wheelchairs. The first kept saying, 'I'm wicked! I'm wicked!' She was obsessed with the fact that she'd stabbed her ex-husband, and no amount of encouragement from me could convince her that God would forgive her. She remained in the chair. The other woman's attitude was very different. She looked me straight in the eyes and said, 'I was prayed for by another minister and I took a few steps. I believe I'll be healed.'

'I'm sure you will,' I agreed. And a few minutes later she was walking around much more, putting her faith into action.

Some sick people have come to us initially more out of desperation than in faith. Perhaps, like the woman with the haemorrhage who touched the hem of Jesus' garment and caused him to ask, 'Who touched my clothes?' (Mk 5:30), they have put their faith in others but have found no satisfactory result. She'd been under many doctors 'yet instead of getting better she grew worse' (Mk 5:26). The very fact that they approach us, though, can mark the beginning of a life of faith for them as we introduce them to Jesus.

Sometimes when we minister healing of body or mind a person may improve or be cured without personally exercising any faith in Christ. But when possible he should be encouraged to trust the Lord as best he can. It's essential that someone trusts Jesus for that person's healing if prayer is used, just as the Canaanite woman had faith for her daughter (Mt 15:28).

Occasionally at our meetings I invite people to claim their healing, but I always add, 'If you feel able to.' Some people have an inability to receive their physical healing until they've first been healed of inner hurts and wounds. They are too sore inside to receive much help in one meeting. And if we suggest they should claim their healing instantly or that it must be their lack of faith which is a barrier, our attitude can leave such folk feeling guilty or rejected.

Where we suspect unbelief we must be careful not to make assumptions. It's not necessarily lack of faith that causes a person to keep seeing his doctor after receiving healing ministry, or to keep taking tablets, or to return several times for prayer. The necessity of these actions all depend on the situation. However, we can encourage people to apply Oral Roberts' three principles of seed-faith whenever possible; begin believing that God will supply all the need; begin giving, knowing that he'll give back to you; and expect a miracle.

How is faith exercised?

BY REACHING OUT TO JESUS

When Chris and I minister healing we constantly point people to Jesus and help them turn their eyes upon him. In the home situation we usually come behind the person we're ministering to so as to help him forget about us and think of the Lord laying hands on him.

Pointing people to Jesus is more than saying 'have faith'. If I say, 'My faith has helped me,' I may be putting my trust in my faith rather than in my God and perhaps even suggesting that my faith used God.

Faith healing is not the same as Christian healing, for many faith healers require people to put their faith in something but not necessarily in the Lord. While we all need to have confidence in ourselves and to trust those who seek to help us, the most important kind of trust in Christian healing is faith in Christ.

Some faith healers also have associations with spiritism, and dabbling in occult practices is dangerous. Chris and I have had to help many people whose spiritual and emotional lives have been in a terrible mess on account of spiritism, as evil forces have inhabited or oppressed them. These people have dabbled in activities like mediumship, séances and fortune-telling which are things the Bible says the Lord detests (Deut 18:10–12).

Who, then, is going to help needy people reach out by faith to Jesus? Ministers are often aware that they are only scratching the surface of the healing ministry.

'How are you, Mrs Jones?' asks the clergyman as he shakes hands with a woman after the Sunday morning service.

'Very well, thank you, Vicar.'

But the vicar knows that Mrs Jones is really carrying a heavy burden—the worry of a chronic sickness which is gradually incapacitating her.

'How are you, Mr Brown?' asks the minister as he shakes hands with one of his deacons.

'Fine, thank you, Pastor.'

But the pastor is aware that Mr Brown is far from fine. He's just become unemployed and is extremely worried because, at his age, he can see no prospect of ever finding work again.

The ministers will probably do what they can for Mrs Jones and Mr Brown, but such people will only find real help and healing as more Christians spend more time with them: listening, ministering, and helping them give their problems over to the Lord.

This ministry is needed for another reason. When someone is sick it's hard for him to muster faith. When I suffered from depression I was often too weak or too tired to pray for myself and became more dependent on the faith and prayers of others. My fears and anxieties had become so exaggerated that they had swamped my faith, but with the aid of caring Christians I came to the point where I could reach out again to Jesus.

Something Chris and I do is encourage needy people to reach out by 'practising the presence of Jesus'. If you can imagine Jesus with you whatever you're doing, this can make a tremendous difference to your circumstances.

Yvette is a young woman who came to us for ministry because she was suffering from depression. Her immediate problem was a violent husband who quickly flew into rages. After ministering to Yvette we encouraged her to go home and practise the presence of Jesus there.

'We've prayed for your protection,' I reminded her, 'now try to picture Jesus with you in that home, and when your husband next loses his temper try to see Jesus standing between you.'

It's this combination of faith and imagination that has so often led to the Lord transforming someone's circumstances.

Sometimes a person is inwardly pained by the memory of an incident in his past. In this case we ask Jesus to go back to the scene of the incident. At the same time we encourage the person to relive the scene using faith and imagination and to see Jesus standing there and putting things right. In this way the sufferer is freed from his hurt and can look back to the incident without further pain.

BY TAKING HOLD OF JESUS

Once we have reached out to Jesus, we must go on to take hold of him. Although the woman who touched his garment did so hesitantly, it was a definite act of trust on her part. She didn't have to work up faith, for it's the gift of God (Eph 2:8).

Putting your trust in Christ doesn't mean trying hard to overcome your difficulties. Once, while praying with a couple who had bankruptcy problems, I saw a picture of a harmonium, the wheezy sort that needs a lot of effort to play. The Lord was saying that the couple were striving and struggling to overcome their difficulties, whereas what they needed was childlike trust in him. They were making hard work of something that could have been made much easier.

It's not a question of trying to get out of a situation but trusting the Lord in that situation. He will then help us find the way out. Such trust should not be confused with feelings either. Many people Chris and I minister to experience encouraging feelings, like warmth or a sense of floating, but some do not. Healing is not feeling, and complete healing doesn't come as we try to find God with our feelings but as we find him with our faith and firmly take hold of his promises to heal.

Occasionally someone asks, 'Shouldn't I be thankful that others are worse off than I am?' Such a questioner is exercising passive faith, whereas effective faith is active.

A depressed lady at Erith refused to see a psychiatrist, insisting 'No, the Lord will heal me.' But when we ministered we reminded her that the Lord could heal her through a psychiatrist as well as through prayer, and that by seeing one she could be acting out her faith in the Lord. After that she did see one, and soon afterwards was restored.

Monica, whose 'incurable' eyelid disease was eventually healed through our ministry at Rustington, had much improved after several months' sessions. She then exercised active faith by asking her doctor if she could gradually come off antibiotics and steroids—a course of action that's right in certain circumstances. The lady doctor couldn't understand what had happened, but she saw Monica's improvement and granted her request.

Miracles don't usually just happen. It was only when Joshua had marched his army thirteen times around Jericho that the walls fell down (Josh 6:10–20). It was when the ten lepers started walking away from Jesus that they found they were cured (Lk 17:14). And it's as we step out in the faith of what has been prayed for that we begin to see the answer. It's no use someone sitting in his wheelchair and being prayed for unless he's also prepared to try to walk with aid. It's no use my ministering to someone in a wheelchair unless I'm also ready to help him to his feet.

When the woman with the haemorrhage touched Jesus it meant that he touched her too. We've seen that a particular way in which we can still express his touch is through the laying-on-of-hands. This is a point of contact for linking the needy person with the Lord and a powerful means of releasing faith into that person and into the atmosphere, causing healing energy to flow.

Outside a church a notice announced in huge letters 'Great Strawberry Tea'. But someone had tried to cross it out, and underneath had scribbled in tiny letters 'Owing to the scarcity of strawberries prunes will be served instead'. It was some years before it dawned on me that I was offering people prunes when I could have offered them strawberries. As Assistant Chaplain at Worthing Hospital I would chat to the patients, sympathize, and perhaps pray with them, but I never realized then that I had something more to offer—the laying-on-of-hands in Jesus' name. I'm sure the 'prunes' I gave those sick folk were valuable, but I've seen far more people healed since I've been offering 'strawberries' too. And it's happened when I've stepped out in faith.

How is faith increased?

By closeness to Jesus

Jesus was constantly surrounded by crowds of sick people, yet he never caught what they had—they caught what he had. There's something infectious about the presence of Jesus. Keeping close to him means getting to know him as our friend and brother, talking to him, and listening to him when he speaks to us, especially through the Bible and other Christians. Above all it means obeying him.

All our problems are not solved when we put our faith in Christ, but if we keep right with him all other things fall into place, and if we keep close to him we're more likely to trust him when a particular need arises.

BY WHAT WE HEAR

'Faith cometh by hearing, and hearing by the word of God' (Rom 10:17 av).

Sometimes Chris and I give those we minister to promises to claim from Scripture, or through prophecy. As the people listen to these specific words for them they may find themselves believing not only that God can heal them but that he will. We also ensure that we have several testimonies at our healing meetings about the great things God has been doing, so that by the time we minister the laying-on-of-hands we have an expectant congregation.

One thing we're constantly proving is that the Lord always means what he says. Sometimes his words are challenging, such as the time when he rebuked his disciples after he'd stilled the storm on the Sea of Galilee.

'Why are you so afraid?' he asked them. 'Do you still have no faith?' (Mk 4:40). He'd previously said to them, 'Let us go over to the other side' (Mk 4:36), and if they had only trusted his word they would have been less frightened, for they should have known that when Jesus said, 'Let us go over to the other side,' he meant that he would ensure they arrived at the other side.

BY WHAT WE SEE

Paul describes his preaching as accompanied by 'a demonstration of the Spirit's power' (1 Cor 2:4). He didn't depend on all he saw, for he also wrote, 'We live by faith, not by sight' (2 Cor 5:7). But he expected to see signs and wonders confirming his message, and he did.

Once we bring people into situations where they see the Lord at work they begin to catch the faith of Christ. As they see people healed, worshipping the Lord with real sincerity and obviously loving one another, many spectators become participants and begin stepping out in faith themselves. The Lord has opened my own eyes in this way to appreciate new dimensions of life and health, and as my vision has increased so has my expectancy.

People take things seriously when things begin to happen. The more they see the more they expect, and the more they expect the more they receive.

By what we do

Cripples have found that after receiving ministry the more they stand up the more they are able to stand up, and the more they walk the more they are able to walk.

One of Satan's tricks is to recreate the symptoms of a sickness after someone has been healed. But if we take it for granted that God is healing us, and persevere in receiving ministry, the Lord will honour our faith. Depressed people and agrophobics know their healing is likely to come in stages, but if they set themselves goals they can gradually achieve these with the Lord's help and gain confidence to go further. The important thing is to act upon the ministry.

Faith is something positive and active, something we do. As we Christians apply the healing ministry—through touch, anointing with oil, speaking words from God and acting upon them—our faith can grow and more healing can be manifested. As we also step out with Jesus the words, the love, the gifts and all that we need will flow. Even if we feel inadequate we'll find once we've stepped out that all the resources are there. We don't have to reach a certain standard, they are freely given.

In these days the Lord is calling his church to be more

outward looking and outward reaching, and this is extremely important in the field of healing.

Rugby players must look strange to those who don't understand the game. All of a sudden a number of the team huddle closely together, their arms around each other, their heads against their neighbours', looking downwards and inwards. Then equally suddenly those men split apart and go chasing off across the pitch in pursuit of the ball.

In the life of faith there is a place for holy huddles, but there comes a time to leave our Christian brothers and sisters and go off into the world in pursuit of the ministry that the Lord has called us to: a ministry to those in need, at home, at work and elsewhere. It's as we go in faith that our own faith will grow and we'll see more people healed through our prayers.

Suggested reading: Mark 5:24–34.

4

Moving the Mountains with the Mustard Seeds

'God, your Bible says prayer can move mountains. Get rid of that one—it's blocking my view!' The old lady drew the curtains shut and went to bed. Next morning she got up and drew back the curtains. 'Huh!' she muttered, 'still there—just as I thought.'

But she'd forgotten what sort of prayer is needed to move mountains. Jesus said, 'If you have faith as small as a mustard seed, you can say to this mountain, "Move from here to there" and it will move' (Mt 17:20). It's the prayer of faith, not hope, that heals the sick (Jas 5:15). If we expect to see God shift mountains of sickness or difficulty we need to trust the Lord when we pray, even if our faith is extremely small.

How should we pray for the sick?

MAKE IT PERSONAL

Jesus didn't heal people from the seclusion of some heavenly operations room; the ministry he gave them was direct and personal.

The number of people healed through their own prayers

is a tiny fraction compared with those healed through the prayers of others, and healing ministry is most effective when Christians pray not just for a sick person but with him. If we say, 'Jesus used to touch sick people. Would you mind if I lay hands on you while I pray?' the ministry we give can be direct, personal and effective. Sometimes it's humbling for a pastor or doctor to accept ministry from an 'ordinary' believer, but if he doesn't his needs may remain unmet.

The first healing in the Bible came through a believing man: 'Abraham prayed to God, and God healed Abimelech, his wife and his slave girls so they could have children again' (Gen 20:17). It's as we pray believing for specific people and needs that we're most likely to see miracles happen. The more specific we are the more effective the healing often seems to be. Jesus has given us authority to speak to each specific mountain, whether it's terminal cancer, marital break-up or mental depression. Our trouble is that we often walk round a mountain hoping it will shift instead of specifically commanding it to.

Once we've named the problem, however, we've no need to dwell on it in our prayers. If I lay hands on a person's back and tell his pain to depart I may then continue praying and letting the healing power soak in, but I turn my eyes from the pain onto the Lord and his plan for the person.

MAKE IT POSITIVE

There's nothing indefinite about the Lord's command to the fig tree: 'May you never bear fruit again!' (Mt 21:19). He is equally positive about the mountain that needs shifting: 'Go, throw yourself into the sea' (Mt 21:21). Jesus was aware of the power of words, and that what we say we tend to get.

Mentally ill people are not helped if we say to them, 'Snap out of it!' They need positive encouragement. If we use negative words in our prayers it can lower people's spirits. Healing begins to happen when Christians open their mouths and pray positively against specific mountains.

It's not just in what we say, either. There's power in positive thinking. If I visit a seriously ill person in hospital and I'm thinking 'He probably won't pull through,' my attitude could be speeding up that man's deterioration. If instead I approach him with faith and a positive outlook, this can aid his improvement.

If we get into the habit of thinking positively we'll automatically pray positively and see positive results. If we feel weak and useless we need to reverse our mental image and constantly repeat aloud scriptures like 'I can do all things in him who strengthens me' (Phil 4:13 RSV). If we pray with a negative outlook people are likely to see us, but if we pray with a positive attitude they are more likely to see Jesus.

One form of positive praying is to become 'two in agreement'. Sometimes Chris and I join hands and agree together for the healing of a person, a relationship, or some circumstances. We claim Jesus' promise that if two of us are agreed about anything on earth it shall be done in heaven (Mt 18:19).

If we're positive believers we're likely to inspire confidence. People will know if they can trust us, and may ask us to pray for them on other occasions. But it's no use praying for Mary, who's badly crippled, unless we're also prepared if necessary to go to Mary and be ready to help answer our own prayers in practical ways.

PRAY WITH PURPOSE

Some Christians hold back from praying with the sick for fear that nothing will happen, and that consequently the sufferer will be disappointed and those ministering look foolish. But these things only apply if the person is specifically told he'll be healed, and this should only be done when God has made it clear or the Christian ministering manifests a gift of faith, one of the supernatural gifts of the Holy Spirit (1 Cor 12:9). Positive praying doesn't mean offering false hopes. We assure the person in need that Jesus is touching him but we stress that the results are in the hands of God.

On the other hand we don't give up praying when we see nothing obvious happening, for we remember Jesus' words about shifting the mountain: 'It will be done' (Mt 21:21). Again, James writes, 'The earnest . . . prayer of a righteous man makes tremendous power available—dynamic in its working' (Jas 5:16 Amplified Version).

In Mark's account of the cursing of the fig tree the Lord tells his disciples, 'Have faith in God' (Mk 11:22). This could be translated 'Have the faith of God'. In healing prayer this means seeing circumstances as God sees them and believing his words are fulfilled before we've even spoken them. It means praying with expectancy—expecting him to meet needs, work miracles and change lives. A woman had a large tumour on her breast, but she attended a healing service and was so filled with expectancy that by the end of the meeting her tumour had fallen off.

It also helps to visualize the sick person whole. If he's blind we can picture him with eyes wide open taking in the beauty of creation. If he's depressed we can imagine him relaxed and laughing. If he's crippled we can visualize him as the man at the Beautiful Gate of the Temple, 'walking and jumping, and praising God' (Acts 3:8).

Praying with purpose also means that we should be ready to minister at all times. The good Samaritan already had on him the oil and wine required when he bandaged the wounds of the man he found by the roadside (Lk 10:34). But Jesus' disciples were not ready when asked to pray for the epileptic boy, so they couldn't cast out the demon that possessed him. 'Why couldn't we drive it out?'

they asked the Lord (Mk 9:28). He replied, 'This kind can come forth by nothing, but by prayer and fasting' (Mk 9:29 AV). He then delivered the boy, however, without stopping to pray and fast. Could that be because he'd already done this?

It's comparatively easy to pray with the sick in the home situation if we have our Christian loved ones around us, and in the church situation where we have a body of God's people to support us. But only if we keep close to the Lord are we going to be ready to minister in the isolated situation.

The day after we moved back to Tunbridge Wells Chris had her hair permed at a local salon. The girl shampooing her hair kept complaining about a pain in her neck.

'I must have caught it in a draught,' she explained. 'Oh dear, I was hoping to go to a disco tonight with my boyfriend.'

For some while Chris volunteered nothing, but when the girl persisted in bemoaning her trouble my wife eventually said, 'Actually we practise the laying-on-of-hands for healing. Would you like me to minister to you?'

'I wouldn't mind,' replied the girl.

So later on, while Chris was sitting in a chair underneath some lamps as her hair was drying, the girl knelt in front of her and received ministry. Everyone in the hairdresser's stopped to watch.

'What are you doing?' asked the Italian proprietor.

Chris was able to explain, and mentioned how this was what Jesus used to do. The girl's neck was soon better, and whenever we pass that shop now all the staff wave at us enthusiastically.

Pray with praise

When Chris and I are ministering to the sick in a meeting the congregation are usually worshipping the Lord, for this helps keep their eyes on him and to release healing power. We also praise him as we pray with individuals, for part of the prayer of faith is thanking him for the results before we see them. Once the person has been ministered to we encourage him to begin thanking the Lord that his healing has begun, and to take for granted that God will move the mountain completely in his way and time.

Even when it's hard to praise God for our difficult circumstances, we can praise and magnify him for who he is. As we see him in control of our situation, things move into true perspective, and our troubles seem small compared with his greatness. Jeremiah is renowned as a mournful prophet, yet every so often he breaks into a prayer of faith such as Jeremiah 17:14: 'Heal me, O Lord, and I shall be healed; save me and I shall be saved.' The secret of Jeremiah's confidence is then revealed: 'For you are my praise.'

If we pray with praise we can expect God to transform our circumstances. Sometimes he does this instantly. It was while Paul and Silas were praising him in the prison at Philippi that the earthquake happened and they were released (Acts 16:25–26). Similarly, some sick folk are instantly freed from their diseases. At other times God doesn't alter the circumstances completely, but he checks them and they stop getting worse. In the same way physical conditions have stabilized after we've praised him. On still other occasions nothing obvious happens outwardly, but people are given peace and strength to carry them through their times of difficulty.

PRAY PERSISTENTLY

One of Jesus' sayings can be translated, 'Keep on knocking till the door is opened' (Mt 7:7). In practice this means that someone should keep on praying until a particular healing is manifested.

We don't have to beg and plead with God to heal. He knows what's best for us and on occasions, in his sovereignty, he chooses to heal without any co-operation from us. However, if someone is given a specific promise that he will be healed it doesn't mean he should then sit back and leave it all to God. The Lord sometimes promises to reverse a condition, but usually it's with the full co-operation of the needy person.

There is no point in someone who has received ministry proclaiming 'I'm healed,' if he's still hopping around on crutches. But his healing has begun, and he should keep trusting and praying until he's seen the complete answer to his prayer. He may still require medical treatment and regular ministry, and if he perseveres in receiving these it's probably not because he is lacking in faith but because he is using it.

Those ministering need to persevere in prayer too. We give up too easily when we get discouraged. If we run into difficulties we should seek the Holy Spirit's guidance about the next step. Sometimes we ask the Lord about a sick person and then fail to wait for God's reply. Persisting in prayer will also mean looking for his answers to specific questions, especially in the Bible and among the Lord's people.

We need to remember as well that the healing service is like a surgery where Jesus is the doctor. It's open for just an hour or two at a time, and although we pray powerful prayers during this time they generally have to be quite brief ones. Many people need following up after these meetings, perhaps with a course of treatment or a series of counselling sessions. I've found that while I've spent on average between two and five minutes praying for someone in a meeting, I seldom spend less than twenty minutes at a time praying for a sick person in the relaxed surroundings of a home.

All this calls for persistence, yet it is seldom that only one Christian is involved in the whole healing process. He may be just one of many links in God's chain of prayer for a particular person in need, perhaps the first link, or the seventh, or the one privileged to see the end result. The important thing is not to miss out on what God wants us to be doing at any particular time. He's depending on believers to share his healing, so if we would share in the joy of seeing the blessings we must also share in the cost of persistent prayer.

We can do this at home on our own too, for while the sick gain particular benefit from direct ministry, Jesus can also touch them as we intercede in their absence. What frequently happens is that the Lord lays a burden for a specific person on a particular Christian who will then pray for him for a period. After that the Lord lifts the burden and gives it to another brother or sister, the next link in the chain.

PRAY PROGRESSIVELY

Jesus moved his disciples on from contemplating the comparatively small fig tree to praying about the gigantic mountain. In the same way, he wants us to start with praying about headaches and minor pains but then progress to ministering for conditions like multiple sclerosis and terminal cancer. It's much more difficult for many Christians to believe that people with these major illnesses will be cured. The problems seem too big, too complicated.

The secret is to pray a stage at a time. Christians are constantly praying for Northern Ireland, yet I suspect that few of us believe all the problems in that war-torn province will be solved swiftly—they've been around too long. But if we know specific people in Northern Ireland, or particular leaders who need our prayers, we will find it easier and more meaningful to pray for them, and can believe for specific things to happen as a result. What we are doing here is praying within our faith.

The same principle applies when we are faced with a big

physical or emotional problem. First ask yourself, 'What can I believe?' Perhaps you can believe a sick person's pain will disappear, or that he'll get a good night's sleep. So pray about these smaller needs first. When we pray like this the Lord answers our prayers, and consequently our faith may grow a little and we can then pray for something bigger. If we pray step by step like this we may eventually find that we can believe for a person's complete healing, salvation or deliverance, and it soon follows.

Jesus promised to do anything we ask in his name (Jn 14:13), so nothing need be out of range of our prayers. There's always a way to move a mountain; all we need to start with is a mustard seed.

A Christian once had a vision of a man examining a wall. It soon became obvious that the man wished to get to the other side, but the wall was too high, too long and too thick. After examining it unsuccessfully for some time, the man was seen to stop and look up. As he looked up he began to grow taller, and he continued to grow until he could see over the wall. Then with one simple movement he stepped over the wall and left it behind him.

Suggested reading: Matthew 21:14–22.

5

'Pick Up Your Bed and Walk!'

Occasionally someone remarks, 'I have Jesus, what more do I want?' A tiny gnat is resting on a huge watermelon. As he feeds upon it he thinks, 'I have the whole watermelon.' But it will be a long time before that gnat can partake of every part of the watermelon. Every believer can say, 'I have Christ,' but there's so much more in Christ for us to enter into and feed upon (Eph 1:3)

So if we desire to see more people healed, we not only need to be living and praying in faith but moving in faith. On at least two occasions Jesus told a paralysed man to pick up his bed and walk (Mt 9:5–6; Jn 5:8). If we want to see more healings like that, we must start walking in the Spirit (Gal 5:25) and moving forward into realms we've not experienced before.

Entering our inheritance

We don't have to fight to win healing—it's part of the inheritance Christ has won for us on the cross. We can enter by faith into what is already ours and encourage others to do the same.

If I'm facing a difficult situation and I ask God to give me faith, he's not likely to throw me down a packet of faith from heaven. My prayer will be answered as I allow Jesus, who lives in me, to release faith through me. I draw upon the trusting relationship that already exists between us.

Healing ministry is often like peeling the layers of an onion. People usually begin by exposing one layer of themselves to God and to Christians concerned about them. Then, when they are ready to expose a deeper layer, he ministers to them at a deeper level. This can be painful, just as peeling an onion can bring tears to the eyes. But it enables the Lord to set people free in their subconscious minds, and sometimes they can only experience physical healing when they allow him to minister to their underlying hurts and fears in this way.

As we lay hands on a person certain needs are brought to the surface, either as he mentions them or as the Holy Spirit reveals them. These are the matters to be prayed about at that time. Later on we may need to move out in faith again as another layer of needs is exposed. If we ask God to lift negative attitudes from people it's important that we trust him to replace them with positive ones. For resentment we may minister a spirit (an attitude, that is) of forgiveness, for anger a spirit of love, for anxiety one of peace, for guilt assurance.

Sometimes we minister new abilities. If someone has a rigid attitude we can pray for a spirit of flexibility; or, if he finds it difficult to relax, a spirit of relaxation. He will need to enter by faith into what has been prayed for by making use of these abilities, but he will be more free to be himself and to relate to other people in new ways.

Experiencing our dependence

The more we move out in ministering to others the more

we have to depend on the Lord. We depend on God to work even when we don't understand his methods, just as we depend on a surgeon to carry out his operation.

While we're waiting for healing it's easy to become pre-occupied with results—'Did he get a blessing?' 'Does she feel God's peace?' But if instead we focus on our relationship with Jesus, these other things are likely to follow.

It's also natural, when the Lord hasn't healed in the way we'd expected, or when someone young has died, to keep asking why—'Why has it happened to us?' 'Why do we have to suffer?' Although these questions are a normal part of grief, we will experience no lasting peace until we stop asking them and accept what has happened. After my wife's second sister died it was nearly two years before Chris found this peace, in her case through a tangible experience of the Holy Spirit. She still couldn't understand why her sisters had died, but she now had no doubt that Jesus was real and had them in his hands.

The Bible says 'Be still before the Lord and wait patiently for him' (Ps 37:7). It also says 'Fight the good fight of the faith' (1 Tim 6:12). How can we obey both of these apparently contradictory commands? The answer is to wait on the Lord till we've received his instructions, then to put them into practice in the battle. Both are acts of faith, but some of us try to bring healing without listening for directions and others are always waiting but never working.

When Paul was shipwrecked at Malta some of the passengers and crew were able to swim to land, while the others had to get there on planks or on pieces of the ship (Acts 27:44). But, as God had promised (Acts 27:24), every one of them reached safety. Those Christians who are stronger in faith can be like the planks. The weaker ones may need to hold onto them until they can stand on their own feet. Those who are just beginning in healing ministry may be looking for support from those experienced at swimming in the deeper waters. But moving in faith means ultimately depending upon the Lord alone.

Don't wait until all your own needs are met before stepping out in healing ministry. The devil loves to get Christians running round in circles solving their own problems instead of reaching out to others in need. But we can receive ministry ourselves during the same period that we are ministering to others. If something weighs us down we must learn to leave it with the Lord, and not pick it up again after asking him to deal with it. Then we'll be free to minister more effectively.

Entertaining our difficulties

'When all kinds of trials and temptations crowd into your lives, my brothers, don't resent them as intruders, but welcome them as friends! Realise that they come to test your faith' (Jas 1:2–3 Phillips).

James' advice is relevant as we minister healing, for sometimes the Lord allows our faith to be tested so that we become spiritually stronger. As we move out in ministry the devil will also be active in our circumstances, but when he flings doubts and fears at us we'll be able to stand firm if we use faith as a defending shield (Eph 6:16) and we'll suffer no serious harm.

Yet it's fear which often holds us back from laying hands on people: fear of not being able to cope, of offending others, of appearing self-righteous, of the questions we might be asked, and of ridicule. Fear is faith in the wrong thing. It's believing the devil and what he says rather than trusting the Lord and what he says. Faith builds up but fear tears down. If we get filled with the Holy Spirit we'll have the boldness to minister, and if we keep our eyes on Jesus as we pray our fears should vanish.

However, some of us Christians, as well as some people who ask us for ministry, have deep-rooted fears. These underlie the way people act and react, so they may need others to minister to them God's perfect love which drives out fear (1 Jn 4:18).

Some are afraid of death, or dying. They needn't be ashamed of this, as Christians sometimes are, because frequently there's a genuine reason in their past circumstances which has caused the problem. The root cause of this fear may be traced back to when the person was in his mother's womb. If a pregnant woman is particularly fearful her anxieties may affect her unborn child, who then subconsciously views the unknown factor of birth as something to be feared. It means leaving the warm and cosy surroundings of the mother's womb. After the child is born he soon forgets the trauma of birth—at a conscious level at any rate. But when he grows older the unknown factor of death may become something to be feared too.

One way we can minister to a person like this is to ask Jesus to go back to when the sufferer was an unborn child and to minister at the root of the problem. If the person being prayed with pictures Jesus calming his fears and those of his mother during the period of pregnancy and birth, and if he trusts the Lord to touch him with his perfect love, he can be set free.

Expecting the impossible

We've seen that one important ingredient in the prayer of faith is expectancy. Another secret of effective healing is maintaining an attitude of expectancy. For many Christians the supernatural has become as real as the natural. This doesn't mean they walk around with their heads in the clouds, but that wherever they are they expect God to do sometimes what no one else can do.

Once Chris and I were at a meeting in Huddersfield and the congregation was singing the song 'Wind, wind, blow on me'. As we sang it a number of us felt a rushing mighty wind enter the room and blow upon us. We were standing in rows at the time and I felt the wind sweeping along our row. It was so powerful that my wife, who was standing next to me at the end of the row, was knocked to the floor.

Why did this happen? I believe it was because that night we were expecting the wind of the Holy Spirit to breathe upon us at that moment. Sometimes he comes more like a gentle breeze, but his supernatural power can be experienced tangibly.

When it comes to healing we shouldn't be surprised if people sometimes receive even more than they expect. The lame man at the Beautiful Gate of the Temple was expecting Peter and John to give him a coin or two, but Peter said, 'Silver or gold I do not have, but what I have I give you. In the name of Jesus Christ of Nazareth, walk' (Acts 3:5–6). Those who've had no tangible experience of God's supernatural power tend to be surprised when people are healed through prayer. Those who have felt this power tend to be surprised if people are not healed.

Before I was renewed in the Holy Spirit I believed that God would sometimes do extraordinary things. But only after experiencing this release of power did I believe that he might want to do some of them through me. Jesus once made an astonishing promise, 'Anyone who has faith in me will do what I have been doing' (Jn 14:12). But he added an even more staggering promise, 'He will do even greater things than these.' If we expect to do the 'greater things' the possibilities are mind-boggling.

Exercising the gift of faith

Peter must have been manifesting a gift of faith when he told the lame man to walk (Acts 3:6). There are some situations, especially before instant healings and miracles, where our usual faith in the Lord is insufficient. God imparts the gift of faith because he knows we need a special inrush for these occasions. Sometimes this is necessary

before we pray command prayers, though usually we only
need a little faith to say 'Be healed' if we leave the details
of how it's going to be done to the Lord.

This gift of the Holy Spirit is among the supernatural
ones listed by Paul in 1 Corinthians 12:8–10. It is very
different from mind over matter or the power of suggestion. While these may play a part in healing they are
natural means, whereas the gift of faith is something we
could never produce from our own human resources.
Some Christians are more likely than others to be given
this gift, but when it's in operation they have no doubt
that God is going to do what they are commanding in
Jesus' name, and often that he is going to do it then.

Howard Carter was a Christian in prison. The concrete
ceiling above his head began to leak and he was unable to
move his head because of the constantly dripping water.

'God, stop that water!' he exclaimed. 'I'm going crazy!'

Back came the reply, 'You stop it.'

'But how can I stop it?'

'Speak to it.'

At that moment Carter knew God was going to heal his
circumstances by performing a miracle, and as he spoke
out he had the gift of faith to believe for it. 'Water, I
command you to go into reverse, in the name of Jesus!'

The water receded, from the tip of his nose straight up
to the ceiling. And not one drop ever appeared again
through the crack in the ceiling while he was imprisoned
there.

Paul exhorts believers to 'earnestly desire the spiritual
gifts' (1 Cor 14:1), so we can seek the gift of faith and it
will come as we are ready to use it. This doesn't mean that
every time we notice someone in a wheelchair we tell him
to get up—we need the Holy Spirit's guidance on every
occasion. But if we feel the need of this gift we can ask for
it, and then we may be surprised at what we find ourselves
saying and doing.

Encouraging the people to respond

It was only when Peter encouraged him that the lame man responded to the command to walk—'Taking him by the right hand, he helped him up, and instantly the man's feet and ankles became strong' (Acts 3:7).

Geraldine was a woman healed of heart trouble through an Anglican healing service. But later a lump appeared under her arm and she went forward for ministry at another service. The clergyman who was leading the service asked this worried-looking woman what she wanted prayer for.

'Strength to cope with this,' was the reply.

The minister laid hands on Geraldine and asked, 'Are you sure that's all you wish me to pray for?'

'Well, I'd really like to be completely better, of course,' she answered softly.

It's this extra encouragement to trust the Lord for their complete healing that many sick folk require. Some also need reassuring that God loves them, that he wants to heal them, and that he's able to.

At many church services the only opportunity to respond to the message is in following a prayer said by the preacher. While this is helpful to some extent, some people need encouragement to respond immediately in a more active way. Healing services provide this opportunity, for people can be invited to come to the front for the laying-on-of-hands both as a response to the address and also to receive God's healing touch. The appeals I give at our own meetings are neither forced nor prolonged but are gentle encouragements to apply what the Lord has been saying, together with a brief explanation of what we intend to do.

Although we're aware that a few people come for the wrong reason, we make it as easy as possible for members of the congregation to come forward. It's easiest for most if we're all standing and singing, and if counsellors and stewards come forward first this gives others confidence to take the plunge. Even so, there are usually one or two people who feel their feet glued to the floor. But if the Lord particularly wants them to come for ministry he may give someone a word of knowledge encouraging them to move forward and receive his touch.

When sick people are unable to get to our meetings they sometimes purchase our cassettes, and after listening to one they release their faith in Jesus by putting a hand on the cassette and find blessing. A lady at Eastbourne who had shingles placed one of our cassettes against her body and trusted Jesus to heal her and he did. Obviously her faith was in Jesus, not an inanimate object, but the act of touching that object in the context of faith actually brought about the change that was needed.

At our training days Chris and I lay hands on few people ourselves. Instead we encourage those who desire to minister to pray with people near them or with others to whom the Lord directs them. Some folk lay hands with others on someone while just one person prays aloud. In this way Christians gain confidence to minister to one another.

Let's encourage those who need healing to use every good means God has provided: prayer, sacrament, medicine, balanced lifestyle, healthy environment, wholesome diet, adequate exercise, and everything else that makes for wholeness. Let's encourage those who minister healing to enthuse about what Jesus is doing and to invite people to see it in action, not just to hear about it at second-hand. But above all, let's encourage them to move out by trusting the Lord to use them in new ways.

Chris has for many years used the word of knowledge in personal counselling and ministry, but one day she asked the Lord for this gift in public meetings (1 Cor 12:8). He soon put her into a situation where she needed it. We were leading the first meeting of our house group at Tunbridge Wells. About twenty people were present, many of whom were not known to us personally. Chris heard the Lord saying, 'You're to minister to someone's right foot.'

'Lord,' she thought, 'why do you have to be so specific?'

But she stepped out and shared with the group what had come into her mind.

Immediately a lady named Wendy said, 'I've just come back from America, so no one knows about this, but I've recently had an operation on my right foot and it's not healed over properly.'

Chris hastened to minister to Wendy, and the Lord completed Wendy's treatment through the laying on of hands and prayer. When Chris saw how he had used her in the gift of the word of knowledge she had the confidence to use it again.

We cannot move in faith if we're spiritually paralysed. Jesus is saying to us what we may have to say to others who are physically paralysed: 'Walk.'

Suggested reading: Acts 3:1–16.

Key 2

GOD HAS NEVER STOPPED SPEAKING: THE GUIDANCE OF THE HOLY SPIRIT

6

The Map in the Doctor's Car

A contributor to *Time* magazine once asked how anyone could obey a God who had not spoken for centuries. Fortunately our God is not that silent—in fact he has never stopped speaking. Without the key of his guidance we can waste much time and see few results, but if we follow what he says we find the way prepared and the signs following (Mk 16:20).

When Chris and I lived on a council estate near Huddersfield I called at a neighbour's house to arrange with Heather about preparation for confirmation as she'd expressed interest in this. Another woman happened to be there and she listened as I shared about what the Lord was doing through our ministry. As a result she too joined the confirmation group and soon gave her life to the Lord. I believe it was no accident that she was present in Heather's home at the time I called, for so often we have found that when we've followed the Lord's directions his Spirit has gone ahead of us and prepared the way.

When the doctor is called out urgently it's vital that he knows exactly where to go and the quickest route to get there. If he is unfamiliar with the area he will consult his map rather than trust his guesswork. Christians who minister healing also need to consult a map—they need to know the Lord's plans for a particular situation, rather than minister haphazardly.

How God works in healing

Sometimes God brings us Christians into contact with needy people and we know it's right to offer ministry then. At other times we're not sure and need to ask him first. Sometimes it's right to invite folk to healing services, at other times it's better to put them in touch with counsellors or specialists. Sometimes sick people will approach us, at other times the Lord will send us to their homes. Sometimes what he requires seems logical and sensible, at other times he may tell us to do something apparently foolish. But we can only minister effectively when we're dealing with the people he wants us to be involved with.

So the most important question to ask is: 'Lord, what would *you* have me do?' (Acts 9:6 AV). This can save us from taking on too many cases and from spending too much time discussing what is to be done. God won't normally bring us a particular need until we're ready to deal with it, but we only have his peace when we're doing what he wants.

EVERY CASE IS DIFFERENT

This is a supreme principle in Christian healing. Jesus healed one blind man in front of a crowd (Mk 10:46–52), another he deliberately led away from the crowd (Mk 8:22–26).

The sick person will need to co-operate with God in whatever way he chooses to heal. If someone is trying to lose weight and he asks for ministry he must naturally expect to eat appropriate foods. If someone is tired from constantly overworking, the Lord may wish him to cut down his commitments as well as receiving ministry.

Sometimes after prayer a person may get worse before being restored. On other occasions it may be three days before any obvious improvement is observed. A lady with cancer of the throat had great faith that she would be healed after we had ministered to her, and only three days later her tumour disappeared. Chris and I have many times seen the promise fulfilled 'On the third day he will restore us' (Hos 6:2). But we wouldn't apply this experience or any one particular method to every situation. When a person has been healed through prayer alone we don't assume that if he falls sick again the Lord will heal him in the same way—perhaps the next time he'll have to consult the doctor too.

The principle that every case is different also applies when the Lord guides us to minister. Though he often does this in supernatural ways, we don't expect all his directions to come supernaturally or we shall be limiting him. We don't tell him how to heal in a particular case either, any more than we would tell a surgeon how to perform an operation.

GETTING TO THE ROOT OF THE PROBLEM

Once the Lord has shown us to lay hands on someone we need to make a right diagnosis or we may offer the wrong 'treatment', like anointing with oil a person who needs deliverance. We can discern the real needs and the root cause through: listening, asking questions, using our experience, and sharing the gifts of the Spirit.

Some people have inherited conditions from their parents or ancestors, and need setting free from harmful ties to these. Some folk suffer disease because of shocks or traumas, so they require healing of memories and hurts as well as physical restoration. Other people bring sickness upon themselves through selfishness or negative attitudes, and need forgiveness. Other afflictions are caused by evil forces, especially spirits of infirmity which is what had happened to the woman with the bent back (Lk 13:11–12). Skin complaints and allergies sometimes fall into this category, and if qualified practitioners are unable to diagnose an illness it may prove to be satanic in origin. In some cases there is a combination of causes. When a non-Christian needs deliverance from evil spirits it's best when possible to encourage him to accept Christ first so that after the ministry he won't fear any recurrence of the problem.

Every case must be treated separately and differently, so we need the Holy Spirit's leading to know exactly how and when to pray. It's important that we listen to his voice because if we don't hear what he is saying we won't know what he is doing (Rev 3:22). During the 1980s he has been speaking to many Christians about outreach, and he wants us to share healing outside the churches as well as within them, just as Jesus used to minister in the streets and lanes.

How God guides in healing

God has such an intense desire to speak to his children that he not only guides us during our meetings but wherever we are if we are willing to listen. When Chris and I are talking together he sometimes breaks into our conversation to encourage or direct us.

He will especially guide us Christians as we seek him before we minister and while we're laying hands on people and praying with them. He often speaks in our minds with a still small voice (1 Kings 19:12). The Lord has been speaking to some Christians like this for years but they have believed it was their own thoughts. If we specifically ask him to guide us, then wait upon him as we minister, we can be sure that what comes into our minds at that time—thoughts, words, pictures or impressions—will usually be from his Spirit speaking to us. And if he wishes to say something very important he is likely to keep on bringing it to our attention, perhaps in different ways.

DISCERNING THE DEEPER NEED

What a person shares is not always his real need. Often when someone asks me to pray about a physical affliction I sense there are deeper problems too, and I know that until these are dealt with the person is unlikely to be completely healed. Jesus asked questions like 'How long has he been like this?' (Mk 9:21). As we ask similar ones we can trust him to reveal what lies behind the answers we receive.

There are direct connections between certain physical conditions and negative attitudes. An ulcerated colon frequently indicates hatred of the opposite sex. An alcoholic often tends to have a dominating mother and passive father. Arthritis may be linked with resentment. This doesn't mean that someone suffering from arthritis is necessarily full of bitterness, but he may have subconscious resentment, and we can gently ask him if he has been hurt by anyone in particular. If the answer is 'yes', we can encourage him to forgive aloud the person concerned and receive healing for his hurts. This ministry has often led to the healing of arthritis.

If someone reveals that he has been to a spiritist healer, or if we discern occult involvement, he may need encouragement to renounce this and perhaps receive deliverance too. Spirit guides, ouija boards, horoscopes and superstition are all means of counterfeit guidance, but once they are given over to the Lord we can minister the healing of Jesus.

Maureen had been involved with spiritism but gave her life to Christ. She sought help from our healing ministry but was harassed by evil forces. One night Maureen dreamed that she was travelling on an escalator. Some white-robed figures appeared and pursued her, calling 'We have chosen you.' But she recognized them to be of the enemy, and in her dream said firmly, 'No, I'm a Christian now.' Maureen wasn't troubled in this way any more, and the dream had helped to confirm her decision to follow Jesus and seek healing from him.

GOD SPEAKS IN A VARIETY OF WAYS

God chooses many different ways to guide both those who minister and those who receive healing. Sometimes he may speak through the Scriptures. Lisa, a member of our interdenominational house-group at Tunbridge Wells, had large gallstones diagnosed and was unsure if the Lord would heal her through prayer alone or whether she should have an operation. She had sufficient money for a private operation if necessary, but first she asked Chris and me to pray about what the Lord wanted.

God told me to turn to Exodus 2:6. We have learned that if he specifies one verse we should begin by reading that but perhaps read further. Verses 6–9 speak of an opening up, a nurse, and payment for nursing. I rang Lisa with the suggestion that God was saying, 'You must be opened up and prepared to pay for nursing.' I stressed that it was up to her whether she accepted this as his leading. Lisa did accept it and was overjoyed, believing the Lord had given her clear guidance and would heal her in these ways. This was confirmed when she went into hospital—she discovered she had a Christian surgeon, and he knelt and prayed with her.

On other occasions God guides through conscience, other people, books, spiritual gifts, supernatural revelations, everyday circumstances or the inward witness of the Holy Spirit. But he will never say anything which contradicts what he has already said in the Bible.

The way the Holy Spirit led Paul to bring the gospel into Europe was through closing other doors. He was forbidden to enter two other provinces (Acts 16:6–7), and the whole course of European history might have been different if he had gone into those instead. Eventually it was a vision that led him to enter Macedonia (Acts 16:9).

Sometimes people seem to need 'dramatic' forms of guidance like visions before they can find healing. Albert was a member of our parish church and a shop-steward in a local factory. He was a Christian, and used his mandolin to accompany renewal songs, but in recent months this activity had become more important to him than the Lord.

One morning before going to work Albert was looking for his slippers. When he glanced up he saw in the mirror a vision of the interior of our church with people going forward for the laying-on-of-hands, himself among them. Immediately he realized that God was speaking to him about his music and that he must receive ministry to help get his priorities right. At the first opportunity he did so, and was also instantly healed of a hernia.

Those of us who minister healing will find the Lord just as ready to guide us at every stage if we wait upon him. If as yet you are inexperienced at discerning his voice, or if you are going through a difficult season and finding it hard to receive clear-cut guidance, you can still minister with other Christians who are able to hear the Lord more clearly.

How we can know God guiding us in healing

'If you want to know what God wants you to do, ask him, and he will gladly tell you, for he is always ready to give a generous supply of wisdom to all who ask him; he will not resent it' (Jas 1:5 Living Bible).

Sometimes when presented with a sudden opportunity, as Nehemiah was (Neh 2:4), we can only breathe a quick 'arrow' prayer. But however brief the request, the Lord will guide us if we bother to ask.

KEEP LISTENING TO HIS INSTRUCTIONS

In the counselling situation this means keeping one ear open to the Lord at the same time as the other ear is taking in what the person is sharing. No one makes a good leader until he learns to be led, and if we would lead others into healing we must first be led by Jesus and not try to lead him.

Sometimes we make our search for guidance too complicated. The Lord may be speaking to us through someone close at hand, like our husband or wife, parent or child. But we'll only hear Jesus' voice clearly during healing ministry if we're used to walking and talking with him. As I'm washing up the dishes or driving the car I can enjoy a very real communication with him that keeps me sensitive to his voice when laying hands on the sick.

Christians who receive the most clearcut guidance are usually those who have been consciously filled with the Holy Spirit. But, however real our experience of the Spirit, we cannot live purely on past experience—we have to keep listening for our fresh instructions.

KEEP LOOKING FOR HIS ANSWERS

Chris has cultivated a spiritual awareness such that she sometimes knows whether something is the Lord's leading by the way her enthusiasm for it is fired or dampened. If we cultivate a similar awareness we'll follow the correct course each time we minister healing.

Sometimes the Lord warns us about something we've been unaware of so that we can pray about it. One night Chris and I had retired to bed and were dropping off to sleep when she had a vivid picture of the Queen Mother. This persisted for some time but we couldn't decide what it meant. The next day we learned that the Queen Mother had swallowed a fish bone the previous evening, causing great discomfort and anxiety, and it was some while before the bone had been removed. We realized afterwards that God had been showing us that we should pray for her. Nowadays if a familiar figure is impressed upon our minds, that is what we do.

We all need to be very sure of the Lord's leading over major decisions such as getting married, moving house, taking on a new job, joining or leaving a church or having a serious operation. Before we make a final decision we may require confirmation from several sources. Sometimes we may be led to put out a 'fleece' (Judg 6:36–40)— that is, to ask for a specific sign within a certain period— but we can never bargain with the Lord.

A driving instructor frequently says to his pupil, 'Keep straight on unless I tell you otherwise, and if in doubt hold back.' Paul applies a similar principle to marriage: 'Each one should remain in the situation he was in when God called him' (1 Cor 7:20). The wisest course when we're unsure is to stay where we are until we're absolutely certain about changing direction.

KEEP LEARNING FROM EXPERIENCE

If we absorb what we learn on each occasion we can make use of it on subsequent occasions, as the Holy Spirit reminds us of particular things (Jn 14:26) and as we put our experience into practice.

Many experiences may seem trivial but are in fact important when viewed in the light of what follows. I've learned, for example, never to engage in long conversations with evil spirits; often to try using soaking prayer when someone improves after one or two sessions of ministry; always to encourage a tense person to relax before receiving ministry; and never to think it doesn't matter about praying with elderly people when their sight and hearing are naturally failing.

An eighty-year-old jeweller at Horsham didn't consider himself too old to ask for the laying-on-of-hands for his deafness. After ministry, Jim tested his hearing by the clocks in the jewellery shop and soon discovered a remarkable improvement.

A helpful question to ask yourself is: 'Which areas and gifts have I mainly been used in up to now?' You will need to develop these in particular, and use the experience gained through them. But be open to discovering the next new area or gift that the Lord desires to use you in.

When you run up against a brick wall, or when someone asks you for the kind of ministry that appears to be out of your depth, you may be able to refer the person to more experienced Christians. But don't let lack of experience hold you back from launching out with others in this vital ministry. The Lord is even more willing to teach us than we are to learn, and we have the added encouragement that his map is always accurate and his plans never fail: 'The Lord Almighty has sworn, "Surely, as I have planned, so it will be, and as I have purposed, so it will stand"' (Is 14:24).

Suggested reading: Acts 16:6–18.

7

The Clock in the Doctor's Surgery

The map in the doctor's car is for his own use while the clock in his surgery is primarily for the benefit of people requiring his help. Every so often someone in the waiting-room glances at the clock, aware that he has had to wait longer than expected and so may need to alter his plans.

It can be like that while we're waiting for the Lord to heal. He is seldom in a hurry and we may have to re-arrange our schedules to fit in with his timing.

The right place at the right time

Christians who minister healing need to be where God wants them at any particular time. Otherwise they experience his second best, and someone they should have been with fails to receive the blessing they could have shared. If we rush around endeavouring to help everybody we'll make ourselves ill, but if we follow the Lord's timing we'll see others healed.

WALKING IN THE SPIRIT

Walking in the Spirit doesn't mean doing something considered spiritual. We can pray in the flesh but wash up in the Spirit. We can do the ironing in the Spirit but read our Bibles in the flesh. Walking in the Spirit means being in God's place at God's time and obeying his instructions.

Sometimes God's clock indicates it's time to take a holiday, or to have a change from our usual routine, for a healthy life means a balanced life. Many businesses will not allow their representatives to work for twenty-four hours after a long plane journey because of jetlag. God knew that we would each need one day's rest in seven (Ex 20:8–11), yet we can easily become like Martha who was 'overoccupied and too busy' (Lk 10:40 Amplified Version). Walking in the Spirit means arranging our time to take on only what God desires.

At a meeting Chris and I were leading the Lord spoke through prophecy:

> I've prepared a table before you piled high with gifts and blessings which are all absolutely free. But some of you cannot enjoy these immediately because your hands are too full of other things. First empty your hands of unnecessary and time-consuming commitments which encumber you, then you can partake freely of the gifts which I have provided for you.

This may mean that sometimes we should attend fewer meetings and spend more time with our families. We'll find that as we become more involved in healing ministry we'll need to know when to say to someone, 'Not now.'

Chris and I have learned not to rush to the aid of everyone who asks us for help, even if someone is desperate or suicidal. We seek the Lord about each case and he shows us when to take action. Sometimes we may put a person in touch with a Christian who lives nearer his home, or who can spend longer with him than we can. But if we do visit a home—provided we're walking in the Spirit—the person concerned is always in and always reaps a blessing.

As you keep close to the Lord you'll get to know when

you are doing the right thing. Chris once called at a hairdresser's to make an appointment, but afterwards, as she did her shopping, she grew more and more uneasy about what she had arranged. So strong was the Lord's prompting that she called at the hairdresser's again before returning home to me, and she changed the date of her appointment. When she arrived home I informed her that I had just booked an appointment with my bishop at the exact date and time when she had first arranged to have her hair permed. Since we each needed our car for these trips, we would have had to alter our arrangements if Chris hadn't listened to the Lord's voice within her.

Changing a hair appointment is a little thing, but little things can be important in the Lord's timing. If we're in the right place at the right time a little thing can lead to something much bigger. We call this the doctrine of the spin-off. Lives have been changed and bodies healed because two people have separately followed the Lord's leading and travelled to where they would meet.

WAITING ON THE LORD'S TIMING

If the Lord wants us somewhere he'll get us there at the right time whatever the cost.

One confirmation that we were to move back to the Tunbridge Wells area was that Chris could only find one college in Kent where she could continue her Human Biology course at Advanced level—West Kent College in Tonbridge. But to qualify for this course she would need to be resident in Kent by June 30th 1984. On June 1st, after months of fruitless searching for suitable rented property in the area, another possible house fell through and we were back to square one. For two hours I rang every estate agent we could think of, but again without success. As we then drank coffee and prayed together, Chris and I began to wonder whether somehow we had made a terrible mistake about where the Lord wanted us to live.

But then I remembered that a lady who lived in the very first house we had enquired about worked in an estate agents. When I rang her she gave me the telephone number of an agent I hadn't contacted, who in turn put me in touch with their office at Biggin Hill. We were getting further and further away from the Tunbridge Wells area. However, to our amazement the Biggin Hill estate agent had just one house available by June 30th, and that was in Southborough, between Tonbridge and Tunbridge Wells —the district where Chris originally comes from. The house sounded ideal in every respect except one—the rent seemed extremely high. Dare we ask if it could be lowered?

'It's unlikely,' responded the estate agent when I suggested this over the phone. 'The owners have reduced it once already. But I'll find out.'

During the next hour we prayed about this, and then the agent rang back to say the rent had been reduced again.

The following day we went to look over the house. We were driving along the Tonbridge by-pass and noticed a couple by the side of the road with their car windscreen shattered.

'Thank God that's never happened to us!' Chris remarked.

But five minutes later it did and for three hours we were waiting in a lay-by for a mechanic to come and deal with the problem. We began to wonder if someone didn't want us to move to Tunbridge Wells.

However, we eventually resumed our journey, and all the other arrangements soon slotted into place. We learned that on the very day I had phoned, the owner's wife had just succeeded in obtaining accommodation with her husband in Germany. She had booked a flight at the end of June and wanted tenants in her house before that date. We signed on the dotted line just a week before moving in, with only days to spare before the deadline Chris had been given by the education authorities. The Lord had timed things perfectly after all.

It sometimes seems to us that he does leave things a little late. Martha and Mary must have felt annoyed and frustrated when Jesus didn't come immediately to his friend Lazarus who was sick. Jesus deliberately stayed where he was for another two days (Jn 11:6), by which time Lazarus had died. It wasn't that Jesus didn't love the sisters but that he knew a greater miracle would take place—Lazarus would be raised from the dead (Jn 11:43–44).

Whenever the Lord delays healing he has a good reason. It may be because he wants us or the sick person to do something else first. It's certainly not because he lacks compassion. He always knows best, so if we can trust him to heal in his way and time we should see more healings happen.

WONDERING WHEN TO PRAY

It's always right to pray for a sick person if he's willing and receptive, but when we're to minister and how the healing happens are the Lord's prerogatives.

There are advantages in praying for the sick in a large meeting. The united praise and prayer is usually a prelude to the Lord moving powerfully in healing, so even a person who slips in at the back anonymously can benefit. But there are advantages in private ministry too. It usually allows more time for a person to share about his needs and for us to minister specifically to each one.

We constantly have to be sensitive to what the Lord wants us to do at a certain point in time. Paul says, 'Rejoice with those who rejoice; mourn with those who mourn' (Rom 12:15). Sometimes I've taken a wedding, then gone at once to take a funeral—in each case trying to

enter into the feelings of those involved. In healing ministry there's 'a time to weep and a time to laugh' (Eccles
3:4), 'a time to be silent and a time to speak' (Eccles 3:7).
Sometimes we pray quietly, at other times we shout—just
as Jesus did when he cried, 'Lazarus, come out!' (Jn 11:
43), or as Paul did when he called to the cripple at Lystra,
'Stand up on your feet!' (Acts 14:10).

There's even occasionally 'a time to kill' (Eccles 3:3).
Paul caused Elymas the sorcerer to be struck blind (Acts
13:11). We sometimes curse cancers in the name of Jesus.
More usually it's 'a time to heal' (Eccles 3:3), and we need
to keep watching God's clock so that we'll be ready to
move at his command.

When to move and when to minister

HOW FREQUENTLY SHOULD WE MINISTER?

We believe in the regular ministry of laying-on-of-hands,
but the timing will vary according to the circumstances.
The right time may be when a sick person has faith to be
healed, like the cripple at Lystra (Acts 14:9). On the other
hand Peter didn't wait for such a definite response before
ministering to the lame man at the Beautiful Gate (Acts
3:4–6). The apostle was on his way to a prayer meeting,
but he didn't say, 'We'll remember you during the service.' Sometimes it may be right for us to make such a
promise, but on this occasion Peter was led to minister
immediately.

If Chris and I discern that someone might benefit from
soaking-prayer we like to lay on hands as soon as possible.
While we're still talking about everyday things the healing
power can be flowing through. On other occasions the
Lord gives us a definite 'nudge' when he wants us to begin
ministering. He may anoint us by bathing me in heat or by
taking Chris's breath away. The way he prompts you may
be entirely different. You may experience no physical

sensations, but if you are open to the Spirit's leading he will show you in some way when to begin.

He will also show you, completely or in stages, the order of needs to be prayed about if there are several. Sometimes a person in a queue for ministry at a meeting asks for prayer for so many things that by the time he has finished his list I've forgotten the first item in it. Invariably I say, 'The Lord knows about all these needs, but which one would you like me to pray about now? Which one most concerns you at this time?'

When a person requires both physical and inner healing it's usually best to pray about the inner needs first, so that underlying barriers can be removed and God's healing power can flow through more easily to deal with the physical problems. If the ministry is prolonged, or if it involves deliverance, we take our hands off the person at appropriate points while praying. This may also be necessary because after a while hands weighing on a person's head can feel extremely heavy. If we place our palms—or just our fingertips—very gently, we can keep our hands on a person for quite a long period without any discomfort.

Don't try to dig up underlying needs if a person is not ready to share them, and don't let Satan wear you down by prolonging a session unnecessarily. One of his favourite tricks is to keep Christians awake half the night trying to get rid of evil spirits. While deliverance ministry demands perseverance, we need to discern when to stop for the time being, place those concerned under the protection of the blood of Jesus, and continue the ministry at another time.

Once I was leading a training conference at a guest house in Llandrindod Wells. As we worshipped the Lord a psychiatric nurse with an occult background collapsed on the floor. But it was five minutes before Sunday lunch, and I wasn't going to give Satan the chance to upset all the arrangements for that, so we left the woman there and ministered to her later.

My wife and I always know when to finish ministering. The Lord may put a word into one of our minds, we may feel the power has drained through our hands, or it may be obvious in some other way that it's time to end a session. We can trust Jesus to take care of every little detail. We always put the onus on the sick person when more ministry is required. We leave it to him to let us know if he is willing for this. But in the limited outreach situation, like a one-off healing service, we try to ensure that no one is sent away empty—everyone can receive the touch of Jesus.

HOW FLEXIBLE SHOULD WE BE?

In some churches healing ministry is strictly confined to one regular service, so newcomers might be forgiven for thinking that the only time they can get healed there is on the third Sunday in the month at 6.30 p.m. What is appropriate for one church may not be for another, and we'll only advance when those of us who lead healing services are flexible about when and how we minister. Thorough preparation is needed for healing meetings but we must also be ready for opportunities which just arise.

In Breath Fellowship rallies we usually have the laying-on-of-hands after worship and the message. But at one such meeting we were only a little way into the service when Chris shared that she was seeing a picture of the old woman who lived in a shoe. Olive, a Roman Catholic lady present for the first time, said she thought this referred to her as she had a lot of children and some problems concerning them. As the Lord had put his finger on this we felt we ought to lay hands on Olive immediately, and not wait for the general time of ministry.

Leaders also need to learn what to do if something 'unusual' happens. One Sunday evening Chris and I were ministering at an informal service in a parish church in

Kent. Among those my wife laid hands on was Gwen, a churchwarden's wife, who sank to the floor immediately Chris touched her. Some time later Gwen was still lying there and her arm was held rigidly above her head against the floor. She whispered to me, 'I can't move my arm.' I immediately discerned that an evil spirit was holding it down, and this was confirmed when someone whispered that Gwen's mother had dabbled in the occult and that Gwen herself had worked with spiritists. The moment I got rid of the demon Gwen's arm came away from the floor as though it had been stuck there with glue. I'm sure that if I had ministered in any other way the arm would have remained locked in that position.

The Lord will always show leaders what to do if they ask him, and the more their desires become his the more they will be like clay in his hands, fit and ready to serve him in any situation.

HOW FAR SHOULD WE GET INVOLVED?

The doctor cannot afford to become too emotionally involved with his patients, and we have to learn to 'switch off' once we've ministered to someone. Sometimes we'll need to be careful about who is present with us. Before Jesus raised Jairus's daughter from the dead he put everyone outside except three of his disciples (Mk 5:37), probably because of people's scepticism.

We'll also need to be careful that our time is not stolen by attention-seekers. Depressed and lonely people may especially take advantage of us by keeping us up late at night or unduly on the telephone. The Holy Spirit will show us when it's right to pray over the phone—often a good way to end a conversation—but we'll need to be firm and positive in bringing this type of ministry to a close.

There are those who go from one Christian to another trying to obtain help. If we keep in touch with others who are ministering we'll often know what part—if any—the

Lord wishes us to play.

Waiting on and working with the Lord

Another person who watches the clock in the doctor's surgery is the receptionist. She does three things we need to do if we would minister healing.

FIND TIME TO WEIGH UP THE CIRCUMSTANCES

A good receptionist is relaxed and welcoming yet keeps things moving in the surgery. We need a similar balance. If we rush ahead of God's timing we find people unprepared to receive ministry, but if we lag behind it we miss important opportunities. So we constantly need to weigh things up. Does this person really want to be healed? Is this case as urgent as it sounds? Should I attempt to deal with this situation on my own?

Sometimes it helps to fast, completely or partially. As we do this we can become clearer channels of healing because we will probably be able to give more time to prayer and be more alert to receive the clear-cut guidance we often need. But fasting, too, should be according to God's clock. If he says it's time to fast we'll find it easier and more fruitful than if we decide to do it just because we think it might be helpful (Is 58:6–9).

TAKE TIME TO WAIT ON HIS GUIDANCE

As the receptionist takes patients' medical history notes in to the doctor she must wait for his instructions. She may be capable of giving advice to people in the surgery, but the final word must come from the doctor himself. In a similar way, if we take time to wait on the Lord we'll be able to communicate his words to sick people and not just our advice, however helpful.

Heaven sounds a fairly noisy place, but even there 'there was silence . . . for about half an hour' (Rev 8:1).

In some healing meetings leaders keep things moving so rapidly that they don't give the Lord a chance to speak. The most meaningful silences tend to be the ones which arise during the worship. If leaders are sensitive to the Holy Spirit they will allow these periods to be times of waiting on the Lord in which he may give words or revelations as timely messages to his people. Quiet times at home can have a similar effect, and meditation has sometimes proved as good a cure for colds and flu as medication.

If we don't wait on the Lord it may be because we're impatient, for his timing is different from ours. If he tells us he will do something 'soon' it may be six months or even two years before he does, for 'with the Lord a day is like a thousand years and a thousand years are like a day' (2 Pet 3:8). Someone may be promised that healing will take place in the spring, then become disappointed when spring arrives and no healing materializes. But, if he keeps waiting, trusting and praying, he may see the promise fulfilled in the following spring.

MAKE TIME TO WORK WITH THE DOCTOR

The receptionist can never take the doctor's place, but she does put into practice what she has been given to do and endeavours to work in with his arrangements. So it is with us who are 'God's fellow workers' (2 Cor 6:1).

Working with the Lord means letting him speak but not trying to force an explanation if we don't understand what he is saying. Occasionally the Lord has given me a word for someone and it has made no sense to either of us, so I've suggested that he 'puts it into a box' and doesn't worry about it. Quite often a few days later the message has become clear.

Working with the Lord also involves constant prayer (1 Thess 5:17). This does not mean that we are battling with God to change his mind but that we incline our minds into line with his will so that he can say what he wants to through us.

Working with the Lord may include ministering to unlikely people. Jesus was so intent on following his Father's guidance that he sometimes went into the hills and spent a whole night in prayer (Lk 6:12). After one such night he took his disciples through a turbulent storm on a lake to a hostile area for the sake of one 'lunatic' who had been banished to the local cemetery (Mk 4:35–5:20).

Working with the Lord means following him whatever the cost, and in the healing ministry it is usually high. However, this ministry is one of great encouragement, for—besides the actual answers to prayer—Jesus provides all the resources we need and never lets us down (1 Thess 5:24). Every so often the Lord gives me a picture of a rainbow, the sign of his faithfulness (Gen 9:16), and I'm reminded that whether I'm in a period of waiting or working his clock will never go wrong.

Suggested reading: John 10:37–11:11.

8

The Thermometer in the Doctor's Bag

When was your temperature last taken? There's a high probability it was when you were ill. One item the doctor may produce from his black bag is a thermometer, for this gives a guide to your progress.

In healing we not only need to consult God's map and watch his clock but also use his thermometer—that is, ascertain our progress. Only the Lord knows this completely, but we can obtain a reasonable idea and the best time to take our spiritual temperature is during a difficult period. When I had my breakdown I realized my faith was not as strong as I had thought, so I repented of a number of things blocking my spiritual progress. My present ministry would probably be less effective if I hadn't faced my weaknesses and surrendered them to God.

To make progress in healing we must keep in step with the Lord. The more contact the sheep have with their shepherd the more they get to know his voice (Jn 10:4). In this chapter we'll look in more detail at some areas of guidance which can help us go forward in healing ministry.

Guidance through the body of Christ

We all need one another, for the Lord's guidance often comes through our Christian brothers and sisters.

LET'S MAKE SURE WE'RE AWARE

Some people may desire to share their problems with us, or seek God's guidance through us, but are too shy to admit this, and we may have to go towards them by offering to pray with them. At the same time we may need healing or guidance ourselves. We each need at least one Christian we can trust and who understands something about our problems.

In everyday circumstances we shouldn't need to consult our church leaders every time we pray for healing, but in church meetings we should only minister under their authority. The Lord can guide as leaders and church members pray and share together, but when Christians are not ministering directly under their leaders they may still have opportunities to bring Jesus' touch to sick people at home, at work, in hospital or elsewhere. Of the forty-four incidents of healing in the New Testament thirty-three occurred outdoors and only eleven indoors.

Healing ministry is most effective when leaders are capable, compassionate, and sensitive to the Spirit's leading. If they listen to constructive suggestions they may obtain a clearer picture of what the Lord desires. At one church where I was Curate-in-charge I preached many times before we decided to hold a short discussion each Sunday morning after the sermon. As I listened to people during these discussions I realized that I had previously been preaching 'above their heads'. Only then did I discover the real questions they were asking.

Something else for leaders to be aware of is the different backgrounds from which people come. Before a bandage is applied to a wound an old bandage may have to be

slowly unravelled; and part of the healing ministry is helping folk unlearn things. If they've been involved with
pseudo-Christian sects they may only find wholeness when
we've helped them lay aside false beliefs and ministered
the truth which sets them free (Jn 8:32).

Leaders in particular can ensure a healing ministry goes
forward in their churches and fellowships. Some keep
their feet on the brakes because they fear offending influential or wealthy church members, but those who encourage the use of healing gifts often see God transforming
lives in powerful ways. Many believers are looking to
leaders for guidance. This means that leaders require constant training so that they in turn can train others to minister the touch of Jesus (2 Tim 2:2).

LET'S MAKE SURE THAT WE SHARE

Among the encouraging signs of spiritual renewal in recent years is a new emphasis on sharing and on every-
member ministry. There's still a place for committees, but
a committee can sometimes be a body of people who take
minutes and waste hours. The place where Christians
often find guidance through sharing is in the small, caring
group.

Once at one of our home groups a lady shared how she
had been looking for a job for a long time without success.
Another lady present was able to tell her about a vacancy
and through this God provided a job for the first woman.
Sharing is sometimes essential when we require confirmation of what the Lord has done. We may need to share
with a doctor to ensure we don't mistake remission or
alleviation of symptoms for a complete cure.

We may need to share with other Christians to ensure
we don't mistake our own desires for God's will. A friend
of ours was leading a service when a man approached him
and declared, 'The Lord has told me to lead this meeting.'

'Well, brother,' our friend replied wisely, 'when the

Lord tells me too you can come up here and lead it.'

The Bible says, 'Test the spirits to see whether they are from God' (1 Jn 4:1). Some questions I ask when I'm not sure if something is truly the Lord's guidance are:

1. Is this glorifying to Jesus?

2. Does it contradict his written word?

3. Is this Christian prepared to submit to others?

4. Does his life generally back up what he says? (Jesus said of false prophets, 'By their fruit you will recognise them' (Mt 7:20).)

Chris and I are privileged to have gifts and talents which complement each other's in our healing ministry. Chris is better in the one-to-one situation whereas I am better at leading meetings. She is better at discerning, and I am better at teaching. Together we discover what the Lord is saying. Sometimes he says things contrary to our expectations, but through sharing with each other and with other Christians we are able to confirm that it is his word.

Once we laid hands on a clergyman's daughter who had cerebral palsy and acute behavioural problems. During the ministry Dawn spoke intelligently for much of the time but intermittently swore at us and uttered deliberately hurtful remarks. We might easily have concluded that this was the result of demonic activity, but we both discerned that it was entirely due to the trouble in her brain. And we were encouraged to learn afterwards that other experienced Christians who had ministered to Dawn had come to the same conclusion.

Healing ministers also need fellowship and ministry themselves. In the midst of so much giving out, Chris and I are grateful for an interdenominational group who regularly minister to us: Christians who seek the Lord's guidance with us and who sometimes pray and fast while we minister to others.

Guidance for the church service

As I've visited churches in different parts of the country, I've discovered some 'ingredients' which the Lord is constantly guiding his people to include when healing is ministered during a service. These are as follows.

THE VALUE OF TEACHING

A church at Shoeburyness held regular teaching sermons on healing in preparation for our meetings there. So many difficulties and misunderstandings arise in this connection that clear scriptural teaching about it is necessary. Many newcomers and their children have had no experience of this ministry, and even those churchgoers who were brought up in Sunday School on stories of Jesus' healing have in the past often heard these explained only in spiritual terms. If preachers expound these accounts applying them to Jesus' work of physical and emotional healing today, this can help answer questions people are asking and also help create a hunger to know more.

One of the best times to minister healing is immediately after the sermon, when people have just been encouraged, taught and challenged about Jesus and the wholeness he provides. This teaching may be followed up at meetings during the week—some house groups use our cassettes to guide them in this.

THE VALUE OF TOGETHERNESS

United prayer and praise from a believing and caring congregation can help release healing energy. The more the people are involved in the ministry the more healing will be seen as a gift for the whole body of Christ and not just the pastor's prerogative.

Some churches include an unstructured period during

their Sunday services when members of their congregations contribute brief prayers, songs or gifts of the Spirit and when the laying-on-of-hands is offered for any need. This can provide an informal 'breather' in what otherwise may be a formal service. The actual ministry may be led by a healing team, appointed by the leaders, who pray individually or in twos with each person who comes forward.

If this is done in the body of the church building it avoids the suggestion that healing is all due to one or two leaders ministering at a distance from the congregation. It may also allow more space if people are overwhelmed by God's power and need others to lower them gently to the floor. And the names of absent sick folk can be read out at appropriate points while the whole congregation unites in prayer for them.

THE VALUE OF TOUCH

British Christians are gradually overcoming their reserve about this. The giving of communion and the ministry of anointing with oil bring churchgoers into close contact with their leaders which may involve touch. The sharing of God's peace is now frequently expressed through hugs and handshakes. But it's again primarily through the laying-on-of-hands that Jesus' healing touch is manifested in church services, and we've seen how vital and effective this can be.

The communion is an appropriate context in which to offer this touch, especially when congregations are not used to healing ministry but are used to going forward to receive the bread and wine. While the communion is itself a healing sacrament, many people also need an opportunity to mention their need and have specific prayer for it with the laying-on-of-hands.

Today the Holy Spirit is guiding many church leaders to make it clear that this ministry is available for any need and that the ministers themselves are simply channels of the healing love and power of Jesus. In the Scriptures laying-on-of-hands is used in connection with penitence (Lev 16:21), assurance (Rev 1:17), healing (Mk 16:18), receiving the Holy Spirit (Acts 8:17), commissioning (Acts 13:3) and specific blessing (Mk 10:16). A blessing is God's grace to help in time of need, and when Jesus laid hands on the children and blessed them we can be sure of one specific blessing some of them would have experienced—any sick among them would have received healing.

Guidance for the healing team

Let me again suggest three important areas which the Lord has been pointing out as worthy of attention.

PRAYERFUL PREPARATION

It's often right to advertise healing services, emphasizing that this ministry will be available. It's usually necessary to discover beforehand the aspect of wholeness God wants us to preach about, together with any specific guidance concerning those we'll be involved with. We also need to prepare ourselves so that as far as possible we'll be clean channels.

POWERFUL MINISTRY

The ministry the team gives will be most effective if each member asks to be filled with the Holy Spirit and doesn't hold back from using the gifts and authority Christ has given him (Mt 10:1). Since the devil hates this ministry, whenever possible Chris and I bind all evil powers from the building before a service—perhaps naming spirits like distraction and confusion—and loose the Holy Spirit's power to glorify Jesus among us (Mt 18:18; Jn 16:14).

PASTORAL CARE

The healing team can play a leading part in the follow-up of those ministered to and keep in touch with them where necessary. While the team is ministering they may sense certain people would benefit from counselling or home visits. If the team meet regularly and report on their progress they can encourage one another and help their fellowships to go forward. To do this follow-up they too will need training. We provide training sessions, seminars and conferences for clergy and ministers and others involved in healing and counselling.

Guidance through the gifts of the Spirit

When Jesus' disciples failed to deliver the epileptic boy he commanded them to bring the boy to him (Mk 9:19). If we get into the habit of bringing sick people to Jesus—both in person and in prayer—we can expect not only definite healing but some direct guidance, and this direct guidance may come through gifts of the Holy Spirit.

ASK THE LORD TO REVEAL THINGS

He can show us exactly what to pray about. Sometimes he does this before we minister. Albert, the same shop-steward who saw a vision of our church in his mirror, had been seriously injured during the second world war. Chris and I ministered to him weekly in his home, often using soaking prayer. Eventually his circulation was going to come back to normal and he would be able to discard the medical corset he had worn since the war.

One evening before going to Albert's home Chris and I were praying together and the Lord gave us a picture of an orange. When we arrived at the house we asked Albert if an orange meant anything to him. Immediately he burst into tears. 'Yes,' he replied eventually. 'It reminds me of when I was in Palestine during the war and I saw a number of my comrades killed all around me.'

By giving us this picture the Lord had shown what he especially wished us to pray about that evening. We ministered to Albert for the painful memories of his time in the Holy Land, encouraging him to imagine Jesus standing there to comfort him. Albert had not even shared many of his experiences with his wife, but after the ministry he was able to recall them without further pain. And, as he benefited from such inner healing, he found it opened the way for his physical healing.

On other occasions it may not be until we're already laying hands on someone that the Lord shows us what to pray about. Felicity was a woman at Horsham who had pain at the base of her spine as the result of a recent fall. Chris placed her hands on the affected part while I prayed, but, as the ministry continued, my wife felt her hands being taken higher up the woman's back until they came to rest upon another section of Felicity's spine.

'No, that's where the trouble is,' Chris announced.

'No, it's not,' retorted the woman, 'the pain's lower down.' But then she added, 'Wait a minute, though. Many years ago when I was a girl of ten I had another fall, and then the pain was higher up where your hands are now.'

Once again the Lord had put his finger on the root cause of a problem.

If we ask the Lord to reveal things he may also expose matters which a person has failed to mention. While ministering to a woman at Crawley my wife had a picture of a news-stand. Only when Chris shared this, turning the revelation (1 Cor 14:26) into a word (or message) of knowledge (1 Cor 12:8), did the woman confess that her husband had been involved in a scandal which had been featured in the *News of the World*.

If we ask the Lord he will show us what more needs to be done. When Chris and I were some way through monthly ministry to another lady, I saw a picture of an unfurnished room. Two of its walls were covered with fresh, clean wallpaper but another was completely bare and the remaining one was partially stripped. The Lord was saying that there were more needs to be uncovered layer by layer before the complete work of healing could take place.

Once the disciples had learnt what they should have done to help the epileptic boy 'they went on from there' (Mk 9:30 rsv). No doubt when faced with other cases of need they would remember what Jesus had taught them. And if we're to go on in using the gifts of the Spirit we must do something more—we must actively respond to the revelations he gives us.

ACT ON WHAT THE LORD SHOWS US

When he guides us through spiritual gifts it may mean we must be ready to minister swiftly. While Chris and I were taking a healing mission in Shropshire I gave a prophecy which stated that the Lord would reveal actual names and addresses of people whom the local Christians were to pray for. At the same time a pastor received a name and address. Soon afterwards he visited the elderly couple concerned, and the following Sunday they attended his church and were converted.

The gifts of the Spirit are available to all believers (Mk 16:17–18; 1 Cor 14:1), and if we really want to progress in the healing ministry we will find we need them more and more as a means of guidance.

Suggested reading: Mark 9:14–29.

Key 3

LOVE: THE KEY TO THE INNER ROOMS

9

The Shortest Man Meets the Greatest

A doctor who had been practising for thirty years declared, 'I've learned that for most ailments the best medicine is love.'

'What if it doesn't work?' he was asked.

'Double the dose,' he replied.

Many people would agree with that doctor that love is a vital key to healing. But what kind of love?

For Christian healing Christian love is the key. The new commandment Jesus gave his disciples was not just to love one another. There would have been nothing particularly new in like-minded Jews enjoying a special bond of love towards each other. What was new was that Jesus told them, 'As I have loved you, so you must love one another' (Jn 13:34). This unique, caring love of Jesus was so different from what the first Christians had been used to that they coined a new word for it—'agape'. And it wasn't long before even their enemies were remarking, 'See how these Christians love one another.'

During the second century A.D. pagan temples of healing required sick people to make offerings, but Irenaeus noted that no fees were charged for healing performed by

Christians. The believers did it out of sheer love for Jesus. Yet this agape love is not something that comes easily, even to experienced ministers of healing. It has to be constantly received from the Lord and channelled towards those who most need it.

Mercy from Jesus

Many sick people need this love but feel too insecure to receive it. Some may not realize that God cares about them as individuals and knows them each by name (Jn 10:3). Others need reminding that Jesus loved ordinary people absolutely and completely, and that he opened his arms to them. We are the ones who can bring that love to them.

WE CAN HELP THEM TO FEEL CHERISHED

Each one of us is unique and more important to God than he is to himself. The Lord cherishes us and he wants us to be ourselves, not what we're expected to be by others. A lady called Tracey shared at one of our meetings how others had caused her to think of herself as ugly, but after receiving inner healing Tracey felt Jesus touch her face with his finger and with that she knew she was attractive. As we pray with such people we often find ourselves loving them with a love we didn't have before, because Jesus is ministering to them through us.

Others, however, almost recoil from receiving the healing love of Jesus because they are haunted by a feeling of unworthiness. Perhaps they've been 'put down' by a dominating parent, or made to feel small by a Christian leader. They can believe God wants to bless them but are so used to thinking they are unworthy that only over a period of time can they receive Jesus' love into their subconscious minds. They may need setting free in Jesus' name from a person who has influenced them, or from a misplaced sense of duty. Such people benefit more from a forgive-ness-centred message than a sin-centred one. They need to know that God doesn't say 'I'll love you when you change,' but 'I love you as you are.'

Over the bed in a prisoner's cell hung a poster stating 'God has never created rubbish.' That prisoner knew that in spite of his crimes he was valuable to God. Like each one of us he was precious to Jesus and worth dying for. The Lord once said to his disciples, 'Don't be afraid; you are worth more than many sparrows' (Mt 10:31).

Lyn was a Christian woman who was worried whether God had accepted her or not because she had let him down so much. He spoke to her through prophecy: 'You're a treasure in my jewel box. You are pure gold to me.'

Some people find healing slow in coming because they are too hard on themselves. Perhaps, like Elijah, they have a low opinion of themselves. When he was depressed and suicidal he cried, 'I am no better than my ancestors' (1 Kings 19:4). The more we help people see how precious they are to Jesus, the more they will accept and respect themselves and so be free to receive his love at deeper levels.

This is his message to each believer. We've no need to grovel like worms once we've received God's forgiveness. We're princes and princesses in his royal family, and we can shout, 'Bold I approach the eternal throne.' Nor need our unworthiness prevent us from being used by the Lord. For he chose Moses—a murderer, David—an adulterer, and Matthew—a thief, to play leading parts in his service.

WE CAN HELP THEM TO FEEL CONFIDENT

A large proportion of hospital beds in this country is taken by mental patients, many of them suffering from guilt. Guilt can stop us from having self-confidence, from be-lieving we're forgiven, from loving ourselves, and from receiving the healing love of Jesus.

A Christian brought up to believe he ought not to have problems may be surprised to find he has more. Not only does he worry about being a burden to others, but he also finds it difficult to live up to what's expected of him. If he feels he shouldn't have resentment he may bury it, but his subconscious mind can only bear so much and the effects may eventually appear in his body. If he harbours guilt about sexual problems he may become obsessed with cleanliness. If he bitterly regrets being a failure he may suffer a nervous breakdown. If instead of holding on to his guilt the believer gives it over to the Lord and shares his problems with understanding Christians, he can experience healing.

Part of the healing ministry is helping such people to regain self-confidence and to know God still loves them. Many will need not only to believe they are forgiven but to be told it and to feel it. A deaconess once confessed, 'I know God's forgiven me, but I can't forgive myself.' She found it difficult because she had a strict father, and so she tended to think of God to some extent as like him. But she was assured through Christian counsellors that God was better than any earthly father, and afterwards she was able to forgive herself. The healing love of Jesus had penetrated her subconscious mind and she was in no doubt that he had forgiven and forgotten.

Many need this reassurance that God not only wipes the slate clean but throws the slate away. Some who doubt their salvation need to be reminded that however much someone fails he always remains his father's son. Others may gain confidence from the 'windscreen wiper' verse— 'If we walk in the light [if we openly share ourselves and our failings before God and before Christians whom we can trust] . . . we have fellowship with one another, and the blood of Jesus . . . purifies us [goes on cleansing us] from all sin' (1 Jn 1:7).

A lady who wondered whether the Lord had removed her resentment was reassured when a man shared a picture of seaweed piled up on the shore and the water nearby clean and pure, showing that Jesus had healed her.

Mixing with all sorts

That lady was a decent, respectable Christian, whereas Zacchaeus was a light-fingered swindler. Is Christian healing possible for people like him? Very much so, for when Jesus spotted the little man in the sycamore tree he had no hesitation in inviting himself to tea with Zacchaeus and his disreputable friends. People muttered, 'He has gone to be the guest of a "sinner"' (Lk 19:7), but on the day the shortest man met the greatest, Jesus brought healing and salvation into that home. The Lord is our example in bringing healing to all kinds of people.

GETTING INVOLVED WITH THE OUTCASTS

We can only share his healing effectively when we're prepared to go towards those who don't naturally attract us as well as those who do. Sometimes in the healing line I'm confronted with a person who could have benefited from a thorough wash before coming, but I remember that Jesus opened his arms to the unlovely. He would not have had any reservations about ministering to divorcees, drug addicts or people of different races. He was set apart from yet thoroughly involved in this world. He managed to maintain a wonderful balance between loving the sinner and hating the sin, and this was no easier for him than for us since he was fully man as well as fully God.

By entering Zacchaeus's house Jesus offended the scribes. We will find that loving as he loves doesn't mean keeping on good terms with everyone. We sometimes need the patience of Job and the wisdom of Solomon, but 'the love of Christ constraineth us' (2 Cor 5:14 AV).

When I was much younger I was extremely shy. I would deliberately walk on the opposite side of the road to avoid meeting people. My extrovert wife encouraged me to go towards others, and people expected me to when I was ordained a minister, but it was only when I was renewed in the Holy Spirit that Jesus gave me a new boldness. I discovered that what I didn't have naturally he could give me supernaturally.

It's possible for Christians to be afraid of getting involved with needy people because of compromising their principles or losing their reputation. But the Lord can use the shyest ones in healing ministry if they really love him and are thirsty for his Spirit (Jn 7:37–39).

In response to the love of Jesus, Zacchaeus offered to repay more money than he had unlawfully pocketed (Lk 19:8). Sometimes it's when people make restitution that they find complete healing. A woman was told she wouldn't be healed until she had written five letters to people she had broken relationships with. At first she was angry and rebellious, but eventually she wrote the letters. It wasn't long afterwards that she was completely healed of mental illness.

GETTING THROUGH TO THE OPPRESSED

Many people are sick or unhappy because they have been rejected or deeply hurt by their parents or others, and some cannot accept forgiveness because they have never really been accepted. Others feel useless because they have never been shown much appreciation, while others cannot give much love because they are unable to receive much. You cannot put water into a broken bottle or love into a broken heart.

But we have good news for the oppressed: 'He heals the brokenhearted and binds up their wounds—curing their pains and sorrows' (Ps 147:3 Amplified Version). Even those who feel numb or dead inside because of some shock they have experienced can find the healing love of Jesus filtering through if we gently minister it to them a little at a time.

Perhaps the best Christians to relate to the bruised and downtrodden are those who have been brokenhearted and rejected themselves. But sometimes the oppressed simply need to feel the touch of Jesus in a tangible way. Every so often Chris and I are asked to minister to someone whose parents were unable to show him physical affection. We encourage the person to give any resentment about this to the Lord, and we set him free in Jesus' name from bondage to his parents. Then, as we pray for healing of hurts, we minister Jesus' touch and ask him to make up to the person what has been lacking. The result has frequently been a tremendous release and a new relationship with the parents.

There are, however, those who are frightened of the loving touch of Jesus; but the Lord has his ways of reassuring them. A pastor's wife knew she needed inner healing but hesitated to come to Chris and me for the laying-on-of-hands because she might fall under God's power—she didn't realize what a lovely experience that can be. But she heard the Lord whispering to her, 'Lean on me,' and then she knew she had nothing to fear.

As for those who can see no way out of their troubles, I sometimes encourage them with Paul's words: 'No temptation [or testing] has seized you except what is common to man. And God is faithful; he will not let you be tempted beyond what you can bear. But when you are tempted, he will also provide a way out so that you can stand up under it' (1 Cor 10:13).

Meeting the deepest needs

Why God allows suffering is a problem which probably prevents more people from putting their faith in him than any other. Because Jesus is a realist he expects us to be troubled. However, he says, 'Set your troubled hearts at rest' (Jn 14:1 NEB). We have to be realistic and admit we've no easy answer to some questions, but we can say that God has proved that he cares by sending Jesus, providing medicine, and answering prayer.

Distressing events in someone's life cause him to become either a bitter person or a better one. Our task is lovingly to minister Jesus to him so that his bitterness dissolves and he is able to face the future with a positive attitude.

PEACE THROUGH PRAYER

After Peter had been through the distressing period of denying Jesus three times in front of a charcoal fire (Jn 18:18–27), the Lord caused him to relive this by asking him three times 'Do you love me?' in front of another charcoal fire (Jn 21:9, 15–17). We can help distressed people associate Jesus with things they would rather forget, so that he can extract the sting from the past and give them peace about the future.

The natural tendency for those of us who are sensitive is to put on masks that disguise our inner feelings. They become a form of protection, rather like a shell, so that sometimes the Lord has gently to break us in order to release his love within us. I believe that is one reason why he allowed my breakdown.

A person at university cannot submit himself for the highest honours until he has graduated through different levels. And our experience is often learning to absorb love at first one level, then another. The more we open ourselves to the Lord the more we enjoy his love and peace.

Sometimes during counselling a person begins by talking about his immediate concerns, but at other times he may start at the commencement of his life. So often the first five years of childhood are significant, and the causes of many problems can be traced back to that period. In naval families a common difficulty is in understanding that God is present, as so often naval children have known their fathers to be away from home.

If someone is so hurt that he cannot remember something, it may not be right to pursue this until it is brought to the surface. Sometimes we may ask the Lord to bring it to the person's remembrance, but he may not always have to picture an incident completely for its harmful effects to be removed. He cannot remember being in his mother's womb, but if the cause of his problems dates from that period we can still encourage him to picture Jesus with his mother at that point in the past.

Alan was a young man who had a terrible fear of dogs because he had been bitten by a dog when aged eighteen. His parents remembered the incident but Alan couldn't— his conscious mind had repressed it. However, he opened his heart to receive ministry and the healing love of Jesus drove out his fears.

CARING AND SHARING

We can see that the healing ministry involves deep and genuine caring and sharing. It also means taking care about whom we invite to minister with us. Imagine how Zacchaeus might have fared if asked to lead a Bible study immediately he had become a Christian. Yet new believers are sometimes given important tasks to do when they have had little Bible teaching or Christian experience. If we love Jesus we will need to ensure, like Peter, that his lambs are fed as well as his sheep (Jn 21:15).

Agape love is not a wishy-washy emotion but a powerful key to healing. One spring Chris and I took several healing missions in the Midlands. In three different churches we all joined hands to sing 'Let there be love shared among us', and each time we did so a woman walked out of the meeting. In one case it was a lady with a spirit of resentment, another had a spirit of rejection and the third a spirit of disruption. The enemy is terrified when Christians unite to express their deep and genuine love.

At another meeting the Lord told the congregation through a prophecy: 'You are like trees that need to be rooted in love.' We are likely to see more people healed as more Christians sink their roots deep into the love of Jesus and draw upon the power of his Spirit.

Love is part of the fruit of the Spirit (Gal 5:22), and fruit takes time to grow. We cannot earn it or work it up but it will arise and develop as we abide in Christ. Jesus said, 'I am the vine; you are the branches. If a man remains in me and I in him, he will bear much fruit; apart from me you can do nothing' (Jn 15:5). As we get to know Jesus in a deeper way we will be able to receive his love in fuller measure, and it will flow through us to minister to the needs of those we pray with.

After he had welcomed Jesus into his home Zacchaeus remained essentially the same little man. When people receive Christ's love they become more free than ever to be themselves. We don't try through healing ministry to squeeze them into a mould of our making. So if someone has been inquisitive by nature he remains inquisitive, but perhaps after the ministry he is inquisitive about different things. The healing love of Jesus can burn out the worst in us and bring out the best in us.

What if it doesn't work? Double the dose.

Suggested reading: Luke 18:35–19:10.

IO

The Patient who Came through the Roof

Healing may be delayed by lack of love. When a Christian moved many miles to a new home he was soon spotted travelling back to his former church. A puzzled friend asked him, 'Why do you still return to your old church when there's one of the same denomination near your new home?'

'I've tried the nearer one,' explained the man, 'but my old church is curing my migraines—that one was giving me them!'

In this chapter we'll look at some areas where love is sometimes lacking and where relationships may need restoring before much physical healing can take place.

Homes of love

When four men brought their paralysed friend for healing they knew that Jesus was in the house because of the crowds which were thronging around it (Mk 2:1-3). People will also get to know if he is at work in our homes. But what can we do when visiting homes where love is lacking?

BRINGING THINGS INTO THE OPEN

We will need to diagnose causes and encourage members of a household to bring them into the open.

One of these causes may be resentful attitudes. It's said that about two-thirds of mental and emotional conditions are rooted in wrong attitudes and about one-third in organic and physical problems.

Negative attitudes like jealousy or self-condemnation can hinder healing, but it's especially resentment that blocks the flow of healing love in our homes. A Christian may try to repress his feelings towards those who are hurting him but this may eventually cause him to be ill or anxious, so resentment needs to be brought into the open and surrendered to Jesus.

Richard was a man suffering from a stomach disorder. When a healing evangelist came to his town Richard received the laying-on-of-hands and felt much better. But about a fortnight later his trouble returned, so he received ministry at another service. Again he appeared to be healed but soon became sick once more. So Richard asked for ministry a third time, and on this occasion he confessed that he bitterly resented his parents and the way they had treated him. He was encouraged to forgive them aloud and received healing for his hurts. Once Richard surrendered his resentment to the Lord he not only felt better but this time the healing of his stomach disorder proved to be permanent.

Resentment can also prevent a person from feeling deeply forgiven, and though he may have inherited a resentful attitude from his parents he is still responsible for it himself as well, and so needs to surrender it to Jesus.

Resentment can also affect how we're used by the Lord. Jonathan Goforth was a missionary in China. During his first thirteen years there not a single convert was known to be won through his ministry. Then he realized he needed to be reconciled to a fellow-missionary whose attitude he resented. Once this reconciliation had taken place Goforth not only lived up to his name but saw many lives transformed.

Repressed anger and grief is another cause which prevents the flow of healing love. Anger and grief are not harmful when rightly directed. Jesus reacted in righteous anger against sickness and stubbornness (Mk 3:5), and against those who turned his house of prayer into a den of robbers (Mt 21:13). John was nicknamed 'Son of Thunder' because of his temper (Mk 3:17), but later became the apostle of love (1 Jn 4:7) and turned his anger on things rather than people—especially things which hurt Jesus (1 Jn 4:1).

So in dealing with anger in the home we may need to remind a person that he can do different things with it. He obviously shouldn't take it out on his wife and children, but should he bottle it up and 'keep a stiff upper lip'? That's what I did when faced with opposition in a church, but it contributed to my breakdown and did just as much harm as if I'd vented my anger on others.

Alternatively, he could release aggression by participating in sport or exercise, and we may need to recommend this. The Christian can also shout at the Lord. The psalmists sometimes threw their anger at him when they didn't understand his ways, possibly shaking their fists at him: 'I say to God my Rock, "Why have you forgotten me? Why must I go about mourning, oppressed by the enemy?"' (Ps 42:9). I don't believe the Lord objected to this reaction. He wants to take our anger upon himself, and we can experience tremendous release if we pour it out aloud to him, possibly in tongues.

Similarly, people need to release their grief. If after losing loved ones they shed no tears they may suffer in body or mind at a later date. The shortest verse in the

Bible tells how the Lord shared the grief of Lazarus' sisters after their brother's death: 'Jesus wept' (Jn 11:35). Sometimes release only comes through tears.

In the Western world men in particular hesitate to express emotion in public. But if they allow us to minister Jesus' healing love to them the Holy Spirit will sometimes cause them to weep and even laugh as they become set free at deeper levels.

BRINGING PEOPLE TOGETHER

When someone becomes a Christian his marriage problems can intensify, especially if his partner doesn't believe in Jesus. Frequently the believing partner asks us to pray about their situation, and he may be the only one we can help in the first instance, but we can minister encouragement and a spirit of wisdom to him.

Harmony between people leads to happiness and stability. The devil loves to split up families, so couples need to make constant adjustments to ensure they are communicating with each other and spending time together. At one time I had to repent of my thoughtlessness because I had put my work as a vicar before my family. While the church family or the Christian community will come high on a believer's list of priorities, the Lord normally wants the natural family to feature even higher. So Christians will wish to show hospitality but be careful about whom they invite to stay with them.

People may require specialized counselling if their problems concern areas like relationships with in-laws, adopted children, or step-parents. But there are two things we can encourage most people to do when they feel able. One is to determine to revive a marriage or relationship and make it much more exciting—variety is the spice of life.

The other is to release to the Lord those relatives who have become a worry to them. Some parents need to allow their children to sin, trusting God to take care of them and bring them back in his time. Others need to stop trying to solve their relatives' problems. Janice was a lady who came to Chris and me in an anxious state because her daughter's husband had left her. At first we could do little to help Janice because she was so worried about her daughter, but eventually we managed to encourage the mother to picture her daughter walking into the arms of Jesus, and to trust him to take care of the situation. Once Janice had done this we were able to minister to her for her anxiety, and a few days later her son-in-law returned to his wife.

Chris and I may encourage a Christian to continue in a home the ministry we have begun. But a person's own relatives are not always the best people to help him as he knows their failings too well, so we may ask the Lord to bring him into contact with someone else.

Jesus is wonderfully reuniting some married couples today. Others remain separated but are given supernatural strength to cope. Others are finding new meaning and depth in their relationship, some discovering that in their cases the best wine has been kept until last (Jn 2:10).

Fellowships of love

Those who minister Christian healing meet with lack of love not only in homes but churches; not only among unbelievers but Christians.

FORGIVENESS INSTEAD OF CRITICISM

When Jesus forgave the sins of the paralysed man the scribes strongly objected to what they regarded as blasphemy (Mk 2:6–7). Their attitude reflects a major obstacle to healing in Christian congregations today—the destructive power of criticism.

Many years ago a pastor kept a complaints book. Beside it lay an old-fashioned pen. Whenever someone in his congregation complained about what another had done he would say, 'Here's my complaints book. I'll write down what you say and you can sign it. Then when I take up the matter officially I'll know how I may expect you to testify.' But the sight of that open book and ready pen caused each one to think again. 'Oh no, I couldn't sign anything like that!' So no entry was made. The minister said he kept the book for forty years and opened it many many times but never wrote a single word in it.

In direct opposition to the destructive power of criticism is the healing power of compassion.

Since Chris and I began our faith ministry in 1979 we have been mainly to churches who desire and expect the sort of ministry we have to offer. But previously we experienced occasions when only some members of a congregation really wanted this, and sometimes there was a critical atmosphere which affected the progress of healing. There were times when we had to 'shake the dust off our feet' (Mt 10:14), for to offer ministry to some churchgoers would have been a waste of time. But there were also occasions when people who at first objected to the ministry changed their minds as Christians involved with us showed them love and understanding.

We have followed a policy of no condemnation, believing that if God doesn't condemn us (Rom 8:1) then we have no right to condemn others. If someone confesses to us a terrible sin, Chris and I obviously don't condone it but neither do we condemn him. And though the Lord frequently speaks through us to such people by his Spirit, we seldom offer advice; we prefer simply to minister the love of Jesus.

So it's compassion which can melt critical hearts, and it's also compassion that aids healing—sympathy is not enough. A mother once brought her sick son to a healing evangelist, but as he prayed she kept making comments like 'My poor boy'. Eventually the evangelist stopped praying and said to her 'Madam, would you mind leaving us for a while? Your sympathy is getting in the way of my prayers.'

GENTLENESS INSTEAD OF DOGMATISM

Leaders also have the delicate task of administering church discipline. Here a secret of healing is speaking the truth in love (Eph 4:15).

Correction has to be applied with caution. We cannot shirk our pastoral responsibility by ignoring arguments that arise among church members, but we need to be gentle when dealing with them. We may have to correct wrong conceptions and misunderstandings, but we will need to do this confidentially and tactfully. If a person is in great pain it's not the best time to tell him his sickness is due to a particular sin he has committed. At that point what he needs most is the gentle touch and loving word which will ease the pain through the power of Jesus.

Communication should be made with care. When a rich young ruler approached the Lord 'Jesus looked at him and loved him' (Mk 10:21). But when the man turned back from following him Jesus neither relaxed his terms nor tried to persuade him to change his mind. Those of us who lead and counsel should cultivate a similar attitude. Like Jesus we may sometimes express humour while ministering, which can help people to relax.

Unlike Jesus we may also need to share openly our personal mistakes and failures. This can help dissuade people from idolizing those of us who have strong personalities or personal magnetism. An early Pentecostal evangelist had a successful ministry and many were converted and healed through him. But one day he stopped appealing in his meetings for people to come to Jesus and invited them instead to come to him. From that moment on his congregations dwindled and his ministry had little effect.

In contrast, when the crowd at Lystra tried to make sacrifices to Paul and Barnabas after a cripple had been healed through them, Paul shouted, 'We too are only men, human like you' (Acts 14:15), and he proceeded to point them to the one true God.

Lives of love

When love is lacking in our individual lives there are two helpful things the Bible exhorts us to do.

WALK IN THE LIGHT (1 Jn 1:7)

This will mean being honest about our needs, our faults and ourselves. There could be no healing for the Laodicean church until they admitted they were 'wretched, pitiful, poor, blind and naked' (Rev 3:17). Sometimes, however, it's not the big sins but the little mistakes that we need to be open about. These are what James is referring to when he writes 'Confess to one another . . . your faults . . . that you may be healed' (Jas 5:16 Amplified Version). Some Christians find it helpful to have one minister or experienced believer they can each bare their hearts to.

In the group context confessing of faults seems best when it arises naturally during a time of sharing or prayer, especially before receiving communion, rather than as an arranged part of the programme. We'll have to be careful if there are people present who cannot easily keep confidences, and we shall not want to hold frequent morbid and inward-looking discussions. But, when directed by the Holy Spirit and able Christian leaders, confession in the presence of other believers can be extremely liberating.

Something which endeared Chris to me long before I married her was her naturalness. And something which grieved Jesus about the scribes and Pharisees was that they were hypocrites (literally 'play-actors'—Mt 23:13).

He had little time for folk who put on a show—he preferred people to be real with him and each other.

A pastor once told me how he prepared to speak about Stephen at his Sunday service but on the Saturday evening felt the subject matter was wrong so prepared an address on Nehemiah. However, when he actually got into the pulpit he found himself speaking on honesty. After the service a young couple told him, 'That sermon was just for us—we've not been honest with each other or the Lord.'

Walking in the light may also mean getting hurt. The more we relate to each other the more we get to know each other's weaknesses, and this can be painful. 'I can trust the Lord,' remarked one Christian, 'it's the pastor and elders of my church I have no confidence in.' People will soon know if they can trust us, and they should be able to if Jesus' love shines through us.

Then there are the pains that arise when we seek deeper Christian unity. Cells in the human body must divide before they can multiply. A man must leave his parents before he can be united to his wife (Mt 19:5). And in the church we sometimes suffer division before we witness unity. But healing of our relationships can ensue as we keep walking in the light.

LAY DOWN YOUR LIVES (1 Jn 3:16)

Notice the lengths to which caring love may go. The four friends of the paralysed man carried him to the house, pushed through the crowd, took him on to the flat roof, made a hole in that roof, and lowered him down to the feet of Jesus, for they recognized the value of the direct ministry the Lord would give him. We're likely to see more people healed when Christians are prepared to go out of their way for Jesus and for those they would bring to him.

For most of us laying down our lives will probably not mean martyrdom, but it will mean falling in love with

Jesus. It will mean following him as a person, not just following his teaching. It will mean seeking to love God with all our heart (our feeling), all our soul (our living), all our strength (our doing) and all our mind (our thinking) (Lk 10:27). It will also mean loving our Christian brothers and sisters, our neighbours and our enemies. The more we appreciate how much the Lord has forgiven us the more we will be able to forgive others. The more we appreciate how much he loves others the more we will love them too. And the more we bring sick and needy people to the very feet of Jesus the more we will see him touch them and make them whole.

If we have received Jesus' love into our hearts we'll want it released through our lives. In the next chapter we'll look at some types of people who desperately need that love, and some ways of sharing it with them.

Suggested reading: Mark 2:1–17.

11

Surprises at the Throne

Jesus' parable of the sheep and the goats (Mt 25:31–46) is one of the many biblical descriptions of healing love in action. In this story the sheep are surprised to discover that by ministering to the king's brothers they have ministered to him, while the goats seem bewildered to learn that by ministering to no one they have failed to meet the needs of the king.

The extent to which we're committed to King Jesus is likely to determine the extent to which we minister in his name to those in need. But which kinds of people most require this ministry?

The hungry and the thirsty

'I was hungry and you gave me something to eat, I was thirsty and you gave me something to drink' (Mt 25:35).

Christians can be in the forefront of those who feed other people's bodies and minds. Many people are also spiritually hungry, not for religion or the church but for reality and for Jesus. If we're to feed them with his love, his words, his gifts and his healing, we and they may need to acquire a 'divine discontent' with what we have had up to now.

Two Indians were sitting beside the river Ganges talking about God. Suddenly one of them ducked his friend's head under the water and held it there for a long time. Eventually the first Indian let the other go and he came up gurgling and spluttering. When he had regained his composure he asked his friend angrily, 'What on earth did you do that for?'

'Well,' replied the other man, 'when you long for God as much as you longed for air while you were under the water, you'll find him.'

Jesus said, 'Blessed are those who hunger and thirst for righteousness, for they will be filled' (Mt 5:6). If this hunger and thirst is not present we can pray that the Holy Spirit will put it there, but our first priority will be to share Jesus with those who are already desperate for caring love.

ATTRACTIVE ADVERTISEMENTS FOR JESUS

It is not just enough to go towards the spiritually hungry. They should feel they can approach us too, so we'll need to draw them by who we are. Jesus said that when we love one another with agape love all men would know that we are his disciples (Jn 13:35).

His desire is that newcomers to our churches will not only appreciate what large congregations we may have or what exemplary lives we may lead but that we are Jesus people. This has been the experience of some folk with no church background who have come into some meetings. Almost before they've heard anything said they've been hit by the love among those present, and drawn as by a magnet to put their trust in Christ.

In ancient times Christians didn't pause to consider whether the Lord would heal, any more than if they should relieve the distress of widows and orphans. They just couldn't help expressing love to people in these ways —it was part of the overflow of the Holy Spirit.

The word 'enthusiasm' comes from the Greek *en theo* meaning 'in God'. The more we discover in Christ the more enthusiastic we're likely to be, and the more we get thrilled with Jesus the more we'll overflow with his love. It's not necessary to have strong personalities for this to happen; if we keep receiving and sharing God's love in everyday life we'll find this flowing through us when we come to minister healing.

A university Christian Union of which I was president was known at one time for its evangelistic zeal and its lack of love. Some of us seemed to be very interested in fishing for souls while forgetting that each fish was a human being needing care and compassion. That attitude began to change as we became more taken up with Christ and lost ourselves in his love.

ACTIVE APPRENTICES OF JESUS

When Paul wrote 'Walk in love' (Eph 5:2 RSV) he meant make progress in love. The best way to do this is to follow Jesus, learn his way of loving, and feed the hungry with his love. But what did he say this would mean?

'If you love me, you will keep my commandments' (Jn 14:15 RSV).

One of the main differences between Christians and others in feeding the hungry is that believers do it out of love for Jesus. We really want to please him, and we may be filled with his compassion for others. However, we don't just feel love. Of course, our ministry would be very cold if it did not include any feeling towards those in need, but Jesus didn't just say to people, 'I love you.' Whenever he was in the presence of sickness he acted, for love, like faith, is something we do.

Jesus threw down another challenge when he said in effect to Peter, 'If you love me, you will feed my lambs'

(Jn 21:15).

In some churches there's a tendency to invite special preachers to adult services but just to ask anyone who might be vaguely interested to teach the children. But Jesus puts the lambs first out of those needing to be fed. Children tend to respond to healing ministry with simple faith but they can soon tell if we think they are less important than adults. It's not just young people who need feeding first but young Christians, whatever their age. Babies need more attention than most people, and so do babes in Christ.

The Lord then goes on, however, to speak of the rest of his sheep (Jn 21:16–17). Believers who have received his love will have a particular concern for other members of his flock, the church.

The night before my graduation ceremony at university I suffered with rampant toothache. It not only affected my mouth but dragged my whole body down and prevented me from getting to sleep. When Paul compared the local church with a human body he wrote, 'If one member suffers, all suffer together' (1 Cor 12:26 RSV). And another part of the healing ministry is sharing in the sorrows of our Christian brothers and sisters while they are undergoing experiences like illness, bereavement, or loss of work. But we may equally find ourselves sharing in their joys, like getting married, having a good holiday, or receiving an encouraging answer to prayer.

Leaders, healers and those in the front-line of God's army also need love, care and regular support in prayer if they are to be built up and kept strong. Those who are new to the gifts of the Spirit will similarly benefit from gentle ministry. We wouldn't wish to be like the group in America who became known as 'The Breathers' because they were always breathing down people's necks. All the flock are capable of digesting the food if it's served up in a thoughtful way.

The strangers and the naked

'I was a stranger and you invited me in, I needed clothes and you clothed me' (Mt 25:35–36).

In the earlier years of my parochial ministry I was sometimes 'taken in' by tramps who called at the parsonage with a request for money. My wife saw through them more quickly, and eventually even I began to question the familiar story-line: 'I've just come out of prison and I've spent all my cash on bus fares.'

Loving strangers doesn't mean opening our arms to every Tom, Dick and Harry who turns up on our doorstep. However, the Lord may call Christians to minister especially to the underprivileged, and there are also many people who are outwardly respectable yet strangers to the Christian faith. Another part of the healing ministry is welcoming such people and spending time sharing Christ's love with them.

THE COST OF DISCIPLESHIP

It means getting alongside them and starting from where they are. When the Good Samaritan saw the wounded man he 'came where he was' (Lk 10:33 AV). When Philip saw the Ethiopian eunuch approaching, the literal meaning of what the Holy Spirit said to the evangelist is 'Go and glue yourself to that chariot' (Acts 8:29).

Suffering people are especially likely to take notice of us if we can say things like 'I've been through what you're going through.' At one meeting a sick man said, 'I've been told I can identify better with others if I remain unhealed. I don't think so, but what do you think?' Chris and I assured him that he could certainly identify with others in his sick condition, but that he would be able to identify just as well after being restored, and could then witness to how the Lord had healed him as well.

But even if we've had little experience of suffering we

can endeavour to put ourselves in the place of the person we're conversing with. Then when we bring him to church, if we Christians each come prepared not just to receive a blessing but to be one, we'll find the stranger feels welcome.

THE CARE OF THE FELLOWSHIP

A congregation is a group of people who meet together, whereas a fellowship is a group who share together. One of the lovely things the Lord is doing in the current renewal is helping his children turn their congregations into fellowships.

A minister was talking to a lady at a sandwich tea. Every so often each of them would pick up a sandwich and bite into it. They were so engrossed in conversation that it was some time before they realized they were both eating the same sandwich. And this is the true nature of fellowship—sharing the same sandwich.

More fellowships are now eating together, spending time together, going out together, and giving even the strangers among them opportunities to share. Although we have to be careful not to spend so much time with the church family that we neglect our natural families, we do want the stranger to feel welcome among us and that he belongs as a person, not just a case; to become part of a body, not a cog in a machine; and above all to experience the love of Jesus:

> I sought my soul but my soul I could not see;
> I sought my God and my God eluded me;
> I sought my brother and I found all three!

When we counsel such people we may have to help them relax, perhaps by first discussing the weather or the latest sports results over a cup of tea or coffee. If during the session the person hesitates to share something because it seems comparatively trivial, we may hasten to assure him that if it's important to him it's important to the Lord and therefore to us. Then after the ministry it may be equally important to put someone at ease. Once when Chris and I had finished ministering I launched into an elaborate spiritual explanation of what had happened. My wife interjected swiftly with 'You do sound pious!' This quickly brought me down to earth again and we all burst out laughing.

However much we make the strangers feel welcome, they will never feel completely at ease if they are conscious of being spiritually naked. Healing ministry may include helping them put on what God has provided for them: 'He has clothed me with the garments of salvation and arrayed me in a robe of righteousness' (Is 61:10).

Jesus also promised his disciples that they would be 'clothed with power from on high' (Lk 24:29). This was fulfilled when on the Day of Pentecost 'all of them were filled with the Holy Spirit and began to speak in other tongues as the Spirit enabled them' (Acts 2:4). Peter explained that 'the promise is for . . . all whom the Lord our God will call' (Acts 2:39). So every believer has a right to these clothes, and is going to be more useful to Jesus if he puts them on.

Suppose a member of parliament walks naked into the House of Commons. He may have an important message to give, but he will lose all credibility with his intended audience. Each Christian has a vital message to share, but if he is to be a more effective witness for Christ he needs to be clothed with the power from on high (Acts 1:8). When we help such a person to be filled with the Spirit, we're also ministering to King Jesus (Mt 25:40).

The sick and the prisoners

'I was sick and you visited Me with help and ministering

care; I was in prison and you came to see Me' (Mt 25:36 Amplified Version).

Let's just take one area of sickness where a release of love is needed for the ministry to be effective.

THE HEALING OF STRESS AND TENSION

An important principle in the healing of this particular condition is 'Let go and let God'.

A violin needs a certain amount of stress, for if its strings are too loose they become floppy and useless, but if they are too taut they snap. Human beings similarly need a certain amount of stress, but when it builds up too much it can be a contributory cause of high blood pressure, migraine headaches, arthritis, ulcers or heart trouble.

Obviously we undergo particular stresses when faced with bereavement, divorce, separation, illness, unemployment or redundancy. But happy times can also be very stressful, such as getting married, moving house, going on holiday or celebrating Christmas. Many of us feel the effects of this tension some months afterwards when we experience symptoms like tightness in the chest, pain at the base of the neck, breathlessness or palpitations. A high proportion of people are on tranquillizers or antidepressants, yet most of them are aware that these tend to ease the strains we are under rather than provide a complete cure.

When Chris and I were praying for one mother with stress problems, the Lord gave us a picture of a big dipper. He was saying that the woman was living on her feelings. She was high while things were going well but very discouraged when bills and worries piled up. We've already seen that healing comes through faith rather than feelings, and Chris and I encouraged our friend to trust the words of the Lord. But when we lay hands on such people we not only pray about the underlying causes and minister God's peace but we also encourage the person to live one day at a time and to take active steps to lead a more balanced life.

Sometimes if people will not deliberately relax God may cause them to stop. 'He makes me lie down in green pastures,' said David (Ps 23:2). Again, Jesus' words in Matthew 11:28 literally mean 'Come to me, all you over-burdened, and I will make you rest.' The healing of stress and tension comes as people 'let go and let God'.

But what about those who have succumbed to stress so much that they suffer from the mental illness of depression? Some of these are restless, anxious and fearful, as I was. Others' minds are confused or weighted down. Others constantly feel extremely low or suicidal. Such folk are accepted more than they were, but there's still wide-spread ignorance about mental illness, and this is especial-ly evident when patients seek to be integrated into the community after leaving psychiatric hospitals.

In addition, Christians are among the many affected. I once heard a radio programme in which the speaker asked, perhaps with tongue in cheek, 'If Jesus healed the mad in mind, why are there so many Christians who are mad in mind?' This made me think, and I jotted down four possible reasons:

1. Because Christians are subject to the same sicknesses as other people.

2. Jesus usually only healed those who bothered to come to him for help.

3. The church doesn't appear to be offering enough heal-ing ministry to its members.

4. Christians are expected to have higher standards than most, and experience particular conflicts when they fail to achieve these standards.

Some believers who are perfectionists also tend to see

everything in black and white, and when depressed seem to desire a spiritual explanation for everything in terms of God's activity or the devil's. But we have good news for the depressed. Since God doesn't want anyone to crawl through life half awake, sick, defeated, tired, nervous and discouraged, he will enable people through healing and counselling ministry to be uplifted, refreshed, restored and strengthened, if they co-operate with him as best they can.

It's often best if more than one Christian or group counsels and ministers to a depressed person so as to spread the load of responsibility over what could prove a lengthy period. We will need to shower him with love, help build up his confidence, then encourage him as he becomes able to surrender his depression to the Lord, think positively, praise Jesus, get fresh air and exercise, and turn his attention to others—a depressed person is frequently self-conscious and inward-looking. At first he may be heavily dependent upon us, but once he starts taking deliberate steps to help himself we may assume more of a supportive role. Encouraged by us, he can find and pursue God's particular plan for his life.

THE FREEING OF THOSE IN PRISON

One other group in need of ministering care are the prisoners. Christians can campaign for the release of the wrongfully imprisoned but are also called to set free in Jesus' name those who have become prisoners of their circumstances.

Many people are imprisoned in their homes. Some are healed through prayer but have to go back into the same environment that brought on their sicknesses. Until that environment is changed their diseases may recur. Other folk have their hands full coping with invalids. Those who look after the depressed and disabled need as much prayer as those they care for.

So do those who cope with young children and the elderly, and so do the elderly themselves. One old lady showed signs of not being on top form and her church-going companions quickly pronounced her senile. They were ready to 'push her down the slippery slope', but caring Christians prayed for her and the result was a diagnosis of diabetes. Once this was brought under control she was her usual self again.

In a later chapter we'll look at the authority Christ has given us to set people free from the attitudes, addictions and influential people that keep them in spiritual, psychological and emotional prisons. Here I would simply recall that the immediate consequence of loving, healing ministry is often a sense of peace, but the result after a few days have elapsed is frequently a sense of freedom. People feel they have been let out of prison and are able to relate to others in new ways.

In all this it's possible to give without loving but not to love without giving. So the next key to healing that we're going to consider seems vitally important.

Suggested reading: Matthew 25:31–46.

Key 4

HEAT, LIGHT AND SOUND: THE GIFTS OF THE HOLY SPIRIT

12

Breaking the Sound Barrier

Whenever there's a power cut, heat, light and sound are likely to be in short supply. It's possible to manage without them for a while but living conditions may soon become restricted and uncomfortable.

The gifts of the Holy Spirit provide heat, light and sound for the church. Chris and I would find it extremely difficult to minister without these gifts. We'd see less power and feel restricted as God's channels.

I'm referring especially to the supernatural or charismatic gifts which I mentioned in an earlier chapter and which Paul lists in 1 Corinthians 12:8–10: prophecy, tongues and their interpretation (sound gifts); words of knowledge and wisdom and discerning of spirits (gifts which throw light on a situation); and faith, healing and working of miracles (heat or action gifts). The Greek word *charismata,* used to describe them, simply means gifts of grace.

Gifts of grace

THE VALUE OF THE GIFTS

The charismatic gifts are pleasing to God. Every gift of God is good (Jas 1:17), and these nine operate as God himself determines (1 Cor 12:11). They especially help to build up his church (1 Cor 14:12).

The gifts have practical benefits. One reason why so many sick people have turned to spiritists and cults for healing is that the church has frequently failed to use these gifts. Many people still don't realize that the gifts help to bring health and freedom. The most recorded of these gifts in Scripture is the word of knowledge, and the most important seems to be prophecy (1 Cor 14:1). The most misunderstood is tongues, the most neglected working of miracles, and probably the most needed in this country at the moment discerning of spirits.

The gifts are passed straight on. A riddle I've occasionally put to Christians is 'When is a fruit tree a postman too?' Like most riddles the answer only sounds easy when you've heard it: 'When it's a Christian who manifests both the fruit and gifts of the Holy Spirit.'

The postman is a particularly helpful description of someone sharing these gifts, for they are not possessed by a believer but manifested through him. They are not for the individual Christian to keep to himself but to be passed on to whoever God addresses them to—just as the postman doesn't own the gifts and messages he carries but is simply the agent who delivers them.

The only time in the Bible that Christians are commanded to covet is when Paul tells the Corinthian church 'Covet earnestly the best gifts' (1 Cor 12:31 AV). The best gift is the one needed at any particular time.

THE GIFTS IN WORSHIP

The gifts exalt the Saviour. Where there's openness to the

gifts Jesus tends to become more central, for the gifts point to the giver. And where the gifts are shared wisely, worship has often come alive in a new way, making an ideal setting for healing ministry.

The gifts also equip the leader. Church leaders can use supernatural gifts in connection with functional ones. The evangelist who asks to work miracles will see God confirming his word with signs and wonders (Mk 16:20). The pastor who manifests gifts of healing will find they help build up his flock. The teacher used in prophecy will frequently see God's word getting through to his hearers with fresh power and vitality. Ideally church leaders will find the gifts beneficial in their main services, but if a church isn't ready to accept them on Sundays they can prove a blessing at mid-week praise and prayer meetings.

Sometimes there's a lot of discussion about spiritual gifts but it takes place in a vacuum. The best place to learn about them is in the context of worship where they are manifested. The spiritual gifts can help decentralize the meeting from being around one person. Sympathetic leaders can show they desire to help church members express the gifts, and can especially make use in meetings of those who have previously manifested particular gifts.

THE COST OF THE GIFTS

There is no need to strive for these spiritual gifts, for we cannot earn them—they are free. We don't have to reach a particular stage in our Christian lives before we can receive them. Nor are they a mark of holiness—it's possible to be filled with the Spirit without walking in the Spirit (Gal 5:25), and to manifest his gifts without his fruit (1 Cor 13:1–3). Where there's division among Christians it's not usually caused by the gifts themselves. When spiritual gifts are manifested they expose the quality of the relationships that already exist in churches.

We need continually to be in a position where the gifts

flow out from the Lord through us to others. When Jesus sent out his disciples to preach and heal he added, 'Freely . . . you have received; freely . . . give' (Mt 10:8 Amplified Version). We can only give to the measure we have received. If we keep receiving from the Lord we'll have more to give, and if we keep giving we'll be readier to receive. It's like the Dead Sea and the Sea of Galilee. The Dead Sea gets clogged up with salt because it has no outlets, while the Sea of Galilee has both inlets and outlets. We need to bring to God any blockages in our lives so that his gifts can flow through us to meet the needs of others.

An important principle here is 'use or lose'. If I've been used frequently in a gift but then keep failing to manifest it, it may 'dry up'. Paul's advice to Timothy then becomes relevant if I desire to be used in the gift again: 'Fan into flame the gift of God, which is in you through the laying on of my hands' (2 Tim 1:6).

It is not enough just to receive spiritual gifts. We need to grow in them. Where a fellowship is growing in the gifts there will not be just the same one or two members always sharing them. Some Christians will manifest certain gifts more than others, but God desires us all to seek specific gifts that we have not used before. When people first suggested I might benefit from speaking in tongues I reacted in my ignorance by exclaiming, 'If God wants to give me that gift, he will!' I'd forgotten that when asking for his gift of eternal life I hadn't said, 'If you wish to give it to me, Lord, you will.' His gifts may have to be specifically sought for and personally received.

Success comes in cans, failures in can'ts. When we stop saying, 'I can't do that because it's not my gift,' and start saying, 'I can do everything through him who gives me strength' (Phil 4:13), we will find the gifts just flow.

THE VOCAL GIFTS

In the rest of this chapter we'll look at the 'sound' gifts:

prophecy, tongues and their interpretation. These have proved extremely valuable in all areas of healing ministry.

A woman once determined to commit suicide by throwing herself into the River Maumee in America. But when she arrived at the riverside there was a Christian meeting in progress and God spoke directly to her situation through vocal gifts of the Holy Spirit. As a result she was prevented from taking her life and delivered from a suicidal spirit.

Sometimes people worry that Christians might get involved with these gifts to get themselves worked up, but very rarely have I known them to be characterized by emotionalism. However, when shared in order, freedom and love, they are God's spoken word to specific situations and are bound to affect our emotions. I don't read a moving story to get emotional but I may well be moved as a result of reading one.

When aeroplanes first broke the sound barrier and flew at over 720 miles per hour it was a milestone in history, but today we take supersonic flight for granted. Many Christians feel speaking out in one of these gifts for the first time is a big step to take, but once they've overcome this initial barrier the sharing of the gift becomes a normal part of their worship and witness.

A good place to start is in the small group. If it's a loving, caring group they will forgive you if you make mistakes. God may give you a 'nudge' or you may just know in your heart when to begin speaking. The important thing is not to plan what you are going to say but to start speaking and trust God to give you the words. If you do, you'll find not only that others get blessed but you will too, and you'll be better equipped as a channel of healing.

The gifts of tongues and interpretation

Speaking in tongues is often the first supernatural gift a

Spirit-filled Christian receives (Acts 2:4; Acts 10:44–46; Acts 19:6), and even when Paul writes to a church that's misused this gift he declares, 'I would like every one of you to speak in tongues' (1 Cor 14:5).

TONGUES IN PRIVATE EXPERIENCE

Speaking in tongues in private aids fitness. Soon after a clergyman aged seventy-five began regularly praying in tongues, people told him he looked twenty years younger. For 'he who speaks in a tongue edifies himself' (1 Cor 14:4).

Praying in tongues also has the effect of relieving tension and giving freedom. We were living 250 miles away from my wife's parents when she learned that her younger brother Paul had suddenly and tragically died. That night Chris lay awake shocked and upset. She didn't know what to say to the Lord about it in English so poured it all out in tongues and found a tremendous release. She prayed in tongues all night.

Every so often someone says, 'I've prayed to be baptized in the Holy Spirit and now I feel all choked up inside.' He's probably been filled but not to overflowing, so we recommend the fuller release of tongues. At one time I thought this was only possible for some believers, as Paul asked 'Do all speak in tongues?' (1 Cor 12:30) obviously expecting the answer no. It was only later I realized that when the apostle asked that question he was referring to speaking in tongues in a church meeting, where they need interpreting. The gift is available to all believers.

When we pray in tongues we are speaking directly to God. 'If I pray in a tongue, my spirit prays, but my mind is unfruitful' (1 Cor 14:14). The Holy Spirit prays through my spirit (Rom 8:26), and I don't usually understand what I'm saying in this language I've never learned. So my mind is free to picture the Lord while praising him, or a particular person while praying for him. Many of our prayer partners intercede for the sick in tongues, and many can testify to the difference this makes both to the folk they pray for and their own prayer lives.

Speaking in tongues involves speaking aloud. In the Western world many Christians pray silently when alone, but if we pray aloud more, both in our own languages and tongues, we'll find it easier to concentrate. We'll also not get easily embarrassed at the sound of our own voices in public, and we'll be readier to pray aloud while ministering to the sick.

Some believers know when to speak in tongues because they sense a supernatural movement on their tongue or lips. Others have 'strange' words coming into their minds. Chris gets 'thumped' in the stomach. We have complete control over the gift once we have received the initial infilling (1 Cor 14:32), so whether or not we receive external promptings we can begin to speak of our own volition. It can be compared to a radio. I decide when to switch on and switch off. I can turn up the volume or turn it down. The only thing I have no control over is the programme provided. In speaking in tongues it is the Holy Spirit who provides the programme (Acts 2:4).

The 'dentist's text' is very appropriate here: 'Open wide your mouth and I will fill it' (Ps 81:10). But that doesn't mean like a goldfish. I must begin to speak, and then the words will come. If at first they are only a trickle, then I must persevere until they become a river (Jn 7:37–39). Someone has expressed it like this: 'Put your brain into neutral, your tongue into top gear, and step on the gas.'

TONGUES AS PUBLIC ENCOURAGEMENT

Tongues are a sign of what God is doing. One way a person knows he's been filled with the Spirit, and how others know, is when he speaks in tongues: 'There could be no doubt about it for they heard them speaking in tongues and praising God' (Acts 10:46 Living Bible).

The gift is also a sign to unbelievers (1 Cor 14:22)—
and unbelieving believers. Some folk have been converted as a result of recognizing a particular language while
listening to a tongue unknown to the speaker. The beautiful experience of singing with the spirit (1 Cor 14:15) has
the effect not only of glorifying God and uplifting a congregation but also of releasing healing energy. So Paul
urges, 'Do not forbid speaking in tongues' (1 Cor 14:39),
and: 'Do not put out the Spirit's fire' (1 Thess 5:19).

Tongues are also a sign of what God is saying. It's after
a message in tongues (that is, from God to an individual or
group) that the companion gift of interpretation is necessary (1 Cor 14:13, 27) so that those present can understand the message. This can bring uplift when a meeting is
dead or flat, and encouragement to particular people with
burdens.

A minister was once considering relinquishing his ministry because it had brought with it so many hurts and
worries, but the interpretation of a tongue spoke directly
to him, assuring him of the Lord's faithfulness. He continued his ministry.

Why then do we need the public gift of tongues? Why
not just the interpretation which everyone can understand? The tongue is like a red traffic-light warning us to
stop and listen because God has something important to
say. We then wait in silence for the green light of interpretation to follow. If I have the interpretation immediately the tongue is given I always wait a while in case the
Lord also gives it to someone else, so as to encourage that
person to speak out.

Sometimes, like Belshazzar's writing on the wall (Dan
5:26–28), the interpretation is much longer than the
tongue since it's not a translation but the gist of what God
has to say. Sometimes it's begun by another person in a
different way than I would have begun it, but almost invariably what the Lord has given to me comes somewhere

in what the person says.

A young man was once given an interpretation but was afraid to speak it out. But after he had eventually overcome his fear and uttered the words, he experienced a painless withdrawal from heroin.

TONGUES HAS POWERFUL EFFECTS

The use of tongues maintains the fire of the Holy Spirit. It is said that whenever during a spiritual revival or renewal tongues has been played down, the 'fire' has died down. So it's important to maintain the gift if we wish to see more people healed.

Chris and I find it helpful sometimes to pray in tongues while using soaking prayer, and while visualizing a sick person as whole.

One other powerful effect of this supernatural ability is in dealing with evil powers: 'In my name they will drive out demons; they will speak in new tongues' (Mk 16:17). Sometimes an evil spirit has refused to leave a demon-possessed person when addressed in English, but once we have come against it in a tongue it has quickly departed. At one rally I was ministering to a man with evil spirits when his mother began screaming as the demon in her identified with those which were being cast out of her son (Acts 8:7). Chris hastened to deliver her and commanded the demon to leave in a definite tone of tongue. Afterwards the two women embraced one another as they rejoiced that Jesus had set the mother free.

The important gift of prophecy

This is the only gift of the Spirit that appears in every New Testament list (Rom 12:6; 1 Cor 12:10; 1 Cor 13:2; Eph 4:11). When Paul urges the Corinthians to 'eagerly desire spiritual gifts', he adds, 'especially the gift of prophecy' (1 Cor 14:1). Prophecy is the direct word of God to a specific situation, and is useful in every area of healing.

Prophecy is often needed before evangelism and healing for these to be fully effective which is one reason why the prophet John the Baptist came before the evangelist and healer Jesus Christ (Mt 3:3). One reason why the success of some evangelistic missions doesn't last is because there hasn't been sufficient preparation through speaking and acting upon direct words from God.

PROPHECY HELPS MAKE NEW

Prophecy brings encouragement. I've often been encouraged by words of prophecy which may be very homely and down-to-earth. Once when one of my churches had a number of problems to be straightened out the Lord said, 'I have some ironing to do.' On another occasion when many of us were feeling tired, he said, 'I want you to feel my love tonight. I'm coming to soothe and refresh each of you by dabbing you all over as it were with soft cotton-wool.'

Of the 33,000 promises in Scripture many are prophetic words of encouragement, and no less than 366 times we read, 'Don't be afraid.'

Beryl was a Christian lady concerned that after ten years' prayer her neighbour Sandra was still unconverted. One day Beryl asked the Lord, 'Please give me something to say to Sandra.' Immediately the words 'Don't be afraid' came into Beryl's mind. So she called on Sandra and they chatted about various topics. Eventually Beryl said, 'I believe God wants me to say something to you.'

'Oh?' exclaimed Sandra, 'what's that?'

'Don't be afraid.'

Immediately Sandra burst into tears. 'How did you know?' she demanded. 'Only this morning I received a letter from the hospital saying I'm to have a serious operation, and I'm terribly frightened.'

Beryl shared how the Lord had spoken to her. And that

was how a gift of prophecy led to Sandra's conversion.

Prophecy also brings guidance. We have already seen how ministers of healing can be guided through prophecy, and I have known some meetings where the theme has been completely changed after God has spoken in this way. When one fellowship was unsure how to proceed the Lord said, 'Put your relationships in order first.' Once they knew his agenda they were able to go forward in the Spirit.

Prophetic words may bring challenge. Part of the healing ministry includes speaking out against injustice and corruption in high places (Amos 5:4, 12). We're not to be ashamed of saying, 'Thus says the Lord,' when speaking against evil political or judicial systems.

True prophecy, however, is never all negative. Nor does it generally condemn, even if it gently rebukes. Challenging prophecies usually speak of specific blessings and what we need to do to enjoy them (Deut 28:1, 2).

PROPHECY SHOULD COME TRUE

God always keeps his promises, so the supreme test of prophecy that foretells is whether it comes to pass (Deut 18:22). God may speak in down-to-earth terms, as when he promised one of our house groups 'You'll be flooded with ladies.' That was the case for a while.

Sometimes he's very specific. He told King Hezekiah, 'I have heard your prayer and seen your tears; I will heal you . . . I will add fifteen years to your life' (2 Kings 20:5–6). Occasionally today he promises a specific time for healing, as in the remarkable case of Nita Edwards who was told she would be healed on February 11th 1977 at 3.30 pm—which was exactly when it happened. But we have to be careful about specific events, numbers and dates in prophecy, as Christians sometimes get things wrong and this can be a great blow to the sick person.

One mistake many of us make is to try and work out

how God will fulfil a promise when he's not mentioned how. The Bible tells us to interpret tongues but it nowhere tells us to interpret prophecy. If we're not sure we again need to share, and receive confirmation.

Personal prophecy also sometimes requires testing. It's lovely when the Lord speaks directly to individuals, but some fellowships seem to feel they must have a word for every person present each time they meet. Let's seek the Lord for personal prophecies but not try to force them.

Other prophecies are 'mixed'. A friend of ours who's very enthusiastic for the Lord has sometimes admitted, 'Sorry, those last two sentences were mine.' This is very different from false prophecy (Mt 7:15), and we can easily forgive him. Nor does it mean if someone's personality comes over in the prophecy that the words are not from the Lord. The Gospels reflect the different personalities of their writers but they are each the word of God.

Prophecy may mean you

'You can all prophesy' (1 Cor 14:31). When a young man complained that two others were prophesying outside the tabernacle Moses remarked, 'I wish that all the Lord's people were prophets' (Num 11:26–29). While we may not prophesy with such beautiful or elaborate words as some prophets and prophetesses, any of us Christians may manifest the gift when opportunity arises (1 Cor 14:5).

We can always expect results with prophecy. In the healing ministry most prophecies are gratefully received and some unlock the door to full restoration. But occasionally like Isaiah (Is 6:9–10), or those who first reported Christ's resurrection (Mk 16:9–14), we may be met with buckets of cold water after we have spoken. The important thing is to obey the Lord. Ezekiel, faced with an unlikely congregation of skeletons, writes, 'I prophesied as I was commanded' (Ezek 37:7).

How do we know when to begin prophesying? A good

time to begin in a meeting is when the anointing rests on the whole body of believers present. Often we sense an 'electric' atmosphere in which people are waiting for God to speak. I find that prophesying is just like opening a packet of tissues. I receive a few words in my mind and as I speak them out I'm given a few more, and so on, until it suddenly stops. One man hesitated to speak out when what he had to begin with was 'The owl in the night . . .', but once he stepped out in faith it became a beautiful message from the Lord. Some people think more in words than pictures and vice-versa. The Lord is likely to communicate through us in the way that comes most easily to us.

Sometimes I have a prophecy 'upon' me, and I know I'm to share it at the earliest opportunity, or that it's to be written down and kept for a particular occasion. But most prophecies are for the moment they are given. Occasionally I begin praying and find I'm prophesying, or vice-versa. Prophecy is neither prayer nor preaching but it may be contained in either, and when people are unfamiliar with prophecy they have sometimes thanked me for my 'beautiful prayer'. It's interesting that they always notice something different about it because of its supernatural content.

Every time the New Testament states that Christians were filled with the Spirit it notes that they said something. As more believers today receive God's power and break the sound barrier by using these vocal gifts, we are likely to see more people healed through prayer. And if any of us remain like Arctic rivers, frozen at the mouth, let's remember that Jesus also heals the dumb.

Suggested readings: 1 Corinthians 14:1–5; 13–19; 26–33; 2 Kings 20:1–11.

13
Lighting-up Time

Some Christians have broken the sound barrier but are not yet observing lighting-up time. They manifest the vocal gifts but have little experience of those which throw light on a situation—the words of knowledge and wisdom and the gift of discerning spirits.

Suppose an experienced surgeon had to perform an operation in complete darkness. He could give and receive a certain amount of guidance by conversing with his assistants, but words alone would not be sufficient to guarantee the success of the operation. Similarly, Christian healing can be more effective when God sheds light on a situation through the gifts I've mentioned.

The value of the light gifts

THEY TEND TO SPELL HOPE

In one of my parish fellowships we discussed the question 'Which is the most important and valuable in healing: spoken prayer, laying-on-of-hands or the word of knowledge?' We decided they were all important and valuable, but the most important and valuable was the means God wanted us to use on any particular occasion. When this was a word of knowledge it sometimes had the dramatic effect of pinpointing specific needs and solutions and carried with it the assurance of healing.

THEY AIM TO SPEED HEALING

A psychiatrist may have to spend long hours ploughing through data to find the causes of a problem while the Christian may be given light on it in an instant. Although the light gifts are not an excuse for failing to use our reason and experience, they frequently have the effect of speeding up the natural, God-given processes of healing.

THEY HELP TO SPREAD HOLINESS

The light gifts do not only aid physical and emotional healing. If they were lovingly used more to expose and display what is happening in the churches there would almost certainly be less deceitfulness and more holiness (1 Cor 14:12).

The words of knowledge and wisdom

Supernatural knowledge is the kind we could never attain by natural processes. It may be given us as we are praying or simply out of the blue. It may come in the form of words, pictures, fleeting impressions or other revelations (1 Cor 14:26). Supernatural wisdom is the ability to apply this knowledge, an ability we could never obtain by natural reasoning.

Occasionally these gifts are bestowed on a Christian for his own benefit but usually they are to be shared. They are messages of knowledge and wisdom and to that extent they too are vocal gifts. If the Lord gives me a picture, for example, I begin to describe it, and I frequently find that this leads to specific healing.

UNEARTHING WHAT'S HIDDEN

Sometimes the word of knowledge brings to light significant events which a person may have forgotten, or repressed with his conscious mind. My wife and I were counselling a lady when Chris saw a picture of a little girl by the seashore. When we asked the woman if this meant anything to her she replied, 'Oh, I'd forgotten. When I was a toddler I was swept out to sea and nearly drowned.'

Even when a person has shared practically nothing about his circumstances God can show us through this gift how to pray. Again and again people have said to me after healing ministry, 'What you prayed about was exactly what I needed prayer for.'

Sometimes people deliberately keep quiet about something but God reveals it through a word of knowledge. When Jeroboam's wife disguised herself the Lord showed Ahijah she was approaching and he called out, 'Why this pretence?' (1 Kings 14:4–6). She had the shock of her life.

While we don't go looking for specific sins, God will bring them to light through this gift if necessary, and we can encourage the person to put things right with the Lord and anyone else involved.

LOCATING WHAT'S MISSING

If the police can trace missing persons with the aid of clairvoyants, how much greater is the Lord's ability to track down what's missing through believers using the supernatural knowledge he gives them.

Chris and I have had many experiences of this, not only in meetings but everyday life. Our elder son, Stephen, was once due to take a driving test but told us, 'I can't find my driving licence anywhere. I've searched high and low. Please ask God to show you where it is.'

We did, and into Chris' mind came a picture of a shovel. This led us to our garage where tools are kept. Then I said, 'Have you looked in the car, Stephen? He hadn't, and there was the licence on the car floor by the back seat. Notice that God hadn't told us the exact location but he had given us a clue to the whereabouts of the licence.

UNDERSTANDING WHAT'S HAPPENING

The Lord may throw light on a situation by giving us inner revelations. At one training day we were asked whether evil spirits could be cast out at a distance, bearing in mind the Syro-Phoenician woman's daughter (Mk 7:24–30). I reminded the questioner that Jesus didn't cast out the demon but uttered a word of knowledge, 'The demon has left your daughter' (Mk 7:29).

Every so often Chris has an inner witness about what's happening to someone. Once she asked a friend, 'What's up?' The friend later remarked that she hadn't realized anything was the matter, but then it had all come bursting out with tears.

Sometimes God communicates knowledge to us through our bodies. In a meeting I may have a burning in my knee which indicates that the Lord is touching someone's knee. I speak out this knowledge and encourage the person to respond. As they minister, some Christians see the affected part of a person's body magnified and perhaps a vivid picture of the surgery that God is performing.

But knowledge is often received through common sense and patience. Occasionally someone says to one of us, 'The Lord speaks to you—he'll show you what my trouble is.' But God isn't a puppet on a string, and we mostly learn what's wrong with people by their telling us.

PUTTING OPPONENTS TO SHAME

Anyone who becomes deeply involved in the healing ministry will encounter some opposition, and Jesus was no exception. But he frequently used the word of wisdom to shame his opponents. When they watched to see if he would heal on the sabbath he said, 'Which is lawful on the Sabbath: to do good or to do evil, to save life or to kill?' (Mk 3:4).

The word of wisdom is a gift one can use without realizing it, and we don't have to be naturally clever to manifest it. Paul writes, 'God chose the foolish things of the world to shame the wise' (1 Cor 1:27). So if you think you are foolish you can confound the wise.

PRESENTING OTHERS WITH ANSWERS

Many are looking for wisdom. It's no use just telling a couple with marriage problems that Jesus can help them—they want to know how.

When Solomon had to decide which woman out of two prostitutes was the mother of a child he gave a word of wisdom, 'Bring me a sword . . . Cut the living child in two and give half to one and half to the other. Immediately the true mother was revealed, as she cried 'Don't kill him!' (1 Kings 3:24–26).

Ordinary Christians ministering healing don't expect to be as wise as King Solomon, yet James writes, 'If any of you lacks wisdom, he should ask God . . . and it will be given to him' (Jas 1:5).

POINTING OUT THE WAY

The words of knowledge and wisdom can throw light on so many situations where healing is required. A lady called Lorraine was conducting a court case against Christians who appeared to have wronged her. But she had doubts about this action and asked Chris and me to pray with her.

As we ministered Chris had a tongue, but she stopped in the middle of giving it because she was seeing an intense, brilliant light. At the same time I was seeing a courtroom and documents being torn up. I shared how I had the words 'Write it off!' and 'peaceful settlement'. The light reminded us of how Saul of Tarsus had also been conducting a case against Christians when God stopped him in his tracks (Acts 9:2–3).

Lorraine was in no doubt that the Lord was telling her to drop the case, which she did, trusting him to vindicate her. For a while it looked as if events were moving in the opposite direction, but eventually the revelations proved true and a peaceful settlement ensued.

The vital gift of discerning spirits

WHY DO WE NEED DISCERNMENT?

Firstly, to counteract the counterfeits. No one bothers to counterfeit half-crowns today because it's only worth counterfeiting what's real and valuable. The fact that there are so many counterfeits of spiritual gifts is evidence of the reality and value of the true charismata.

Resurgence of interest in the occult is one reason why we need the supernatural ability to discern which spirit is motivating someone on certain occasions. Many Christians have been mobilized to speak and pray against occult activities but something more is needed. If the church made more use of discernment of spirits we might not see so many people turning to occult healers for reality and comfort. There is a vital need in every fellowship for at least one Christian who regularly manifests this gift. Leaders may be gifted in other ways but lacking in discernment.

We also need discernment to dodge the deceiver. Satan's chief strategy is probably not temptation, oppression or possession but deception. Since he was originally called Lucifer, or light-bearer (Is 14:12; Lk 10:18) he has no difficulty in disguising himself as an angel of light (2 Cor 11:14). Without discernment Christians can easily be taken in by logicality or apparent charm.

When Peter confessed, 'You are the Christ, the Son of the living God,' Jesus discerned that God gave the apostle these words. But a short while afterwards, when Peter said of Christ's impending crucifixion, 'This shall never happen to you!' Jesus retorted, 'Out of my sight, Satan!' Peter's words may sound kind to the unwary listener but they were motivated not by 'the things of God, but the things of men' (Mt 16:16–23).

Sometimes even Christians in leadership can be deceived. After all, if you were the devil wouldn't you want to get your agents into parochial church councils and deacons' meetings?

We need discernment because the enemy can take us by surprise. He is likely to use a different method to deceive us next time than he did last time. However, he has three favourite tactics which he uses frequently with those who minister healing and deliverance. First, he'll blow up little things to make them appear large. Secondly, he'll try to wear down believers by delaying tactics. Thirdly, he'll pretend to hide away in the hope that he and his agents will be ignored. In cases of multiple possession the last demon, which is usually also the strongest, has sometimes succeeded in convincing those ministering that it is nonexistent.

Less frequently the enemy sometimes twists what is said so that someone hears something different from what was spoken—perhaps even the opposite. Satan must use more subtle wiles to deceive more experienced Christians, but they still need razor-sharp discernment.

Thirdly, we need discernment to arm for action.

Anyone who ministers Christian healing must be prepared for some deliverance ministry. However, he is wise not to take the lead in this if it involves exorcism, unless he has had experience in that realm. In the first instance it's best for a Christian to observe what others do and support them in prayer. But all involved need to put on God's armour for the battle (Eph 6:10–18).

WHAT DO WE NEED TO DISCERN?

It is important at the outset that we ask the Lord which spirit is motivating a person—his human spirit, the Holy Spirit or an evil spirit. Sometimes God reveals the type of evil force involved, like a spirit of divination (Acts 16:16) or infirmity (Lk 13:11). It's not always necessary to know this, but it helps in encouraging people to renounce specific activities.

Sometimes it's our selfish natures that get in the way of God's healing work (Rom 8:5–8). Jesus discerned that the Pharisees were blinder than the blind man (Jn 9:41), and Peter sometimes tried to manipulate the Lord (Mt 16:22). We need to discern when people are manipulating us.

Once we have discerned which spirit is motivating a person, then we can seek the Lord for the right solution. If we discover whether a person is motivated by a negative attitude or a demon, we will know whether to minister inner healing or deliverance, whether to pray 'Be healed!' or 'I set you free'.

One man was fifty-two years in a mental hospital diagnosed as schizophrenic. But a Christian psychiatrist discerned that this patient was demon-possessed, and obtained permission to deliver him. The man was released from the hospital, free 'and in his right mind' (Mk 5:15).

We may need to discern in which areas Satan has a hold on someone, and consequently how to minister. Certain Christians who were demon-possessed before they were converted may need deliverance afterwards. When a person is born again his sins are forgiven but he can still fail; he is healed but can still fall sick; and he has left the kingdom of Satan for the kingdom of God but, if the enemy still has a hold on him, he will not always let go until specifically commanded to.

Demons only tend to manifest themselves among Christians when the Lord's power is fully released, just as they cried out in Jesus' real presence when he walked the earth (Mk 3:11). But they didn't automatically flee at his presence, they had to be told to go (Mk 1:23–26).

There's no point in looking for demons, and no need to fear them if we walk with the Lord, but should we Christians discern their presence, we have Jesus' authority to deal with them (Mt 10:1; Mk 16:17). Although Simon the sorcerer believed and was baptized (Acts 8:13), Peter discerned that he was still 'full of bitterness and captive to sin' (Acts 8:23). And though a Christian may have renounced evil and occult involvement, Satan may still have a hold on him in a related area which he has forgotten about, so deliverance may be necessary.

A Christian lady was exorcized at one of our meetings. Afterwards she asked, 'How could I be used in prophecy yet still have evil within me?' I explained that she was only possessed during the period she was taken over by the spirit when it reacted in fear to what God was doing. It was a separate entity within her. She needed to be built up spiritually and be strong to co-operate in any future battle. If the Enemy still had a hold on her she might not be able to break this through her own prayers but might need further ministry from other believers. But most of the time she could lead a normal Christian life and be used by God in whatever gifts he gave her.

HOW ARE WE ABLE TO DISCERN?
The sufferers may reveal symptoms that enlighten us about their condition.

'I became a Christian after your meeting at Hailsham,' a man called Derek told me, 'but however hard I try I just can't seem to pray. I used to dabble in spiritism, but I've renounced that.' As soon as I laid hands on Derek he started shaking all over. Then as I commanded the spirit to leave he slumped to the floor. Afterwards he was rejoicing in the difference Jesus had made to him.

When people are not forthcoming about their background, God may show us through particular ways that he communicates to us that Satan has a hold on them. Chris may be hit by a sense of blackness, I by a feeling of icy feet. A young Christian was travelling on a train when suddenly she felt as though her hair stood up on end. A moment later the man opposite her pulled out of his pocket a book on the occult.

Another Christian was praying with a stranger. He was stumped about the problem concerned, but as he started to pray he suddenly broke out in grief and crying. As a result the stranger opened up, confessed his sins, repented of them, and was set free.

The codes God builds up with you may be entirely different from these, but you can get to know his communication signals.

Sensitivity is always required by those in the deliverance ministry. One way I know while ministering that I'm dealing with a demon is when the word 'daiomonia' creeps into my prayer language. Chris sometimes identifies with the physical sensations experienced by the person ministered to. As evil spirits leave someone she may simultaneously feel as if they are leaving her.

When we ministered to a woman at Crawley, my wife saw some mice pegging out garments on a clothes-line. The Lord was saying that evil forces had specific holds on the woman through hurt, guilt and fear. Our task was to help remove the pegs through ministry in Jesus' name. The Lord often shows us mice when we are dealing with Satan's agents, probably to indicate their smallness against his greatness. Sometimes they carry suitcases, but as we command the demons to leave we see the mice fleeing and dropping their cases, then perhaps disappearing through a trapdoor. Simultaneously we know that evil spirits have departed from the person concerned.

If someone has been to a healer and we are not sure

how helpful he has been, we can set the person free in Jesus' name from any harm that has been done and pray for any discernment needed. When we discern that a headache is not caused by migraine, sinusitis, neuralgia or tension but demonic oppression, that headache will usually disappear instantly on being rebuked.

Being able to detect what others cannot see can prove a lonely experience. Chris and I were once in a rousing charismatic meeting when she whispered, 'There's something terribly wrong here.' Everyone seemed to be thoroughly enjoying themselves but a few weeks later a number of serious problems at that church came to light. Chris had not felt it right to share her misgivings with others, however, as they would probably have rejected them. If we are given discernment it's sometimes right to keep it to ourselves until an appropriate time.

Whether the problems God brings to light are little or vast we have no need to fear, for we are not dealing with two persons of equal strength but with an enemy who has a little power and a God who has tremendous power and who triumphed over all evil forces on the cross (Eph 2:15). So, just as the Israelites claimed God's protection by daubing their doorposts with the blood of the passover lambs (Ex 12:21–23), we can claim the protection of the blood of Jesus. If we do this, and walk in the Spirit, we will not need protection from the Enemy—he will need protection from us. Jesus' victory is assured and permanent, but our need is to observe lighting-up time.

Suggested reading: Mark 7:24–37.

14
Turning on the Heat

The action gifts of faith, healing and miracles are regarded by some Christians as 'too hot to handle', yet they are sometimes the key to spiritual awakening. Jesus said to the Laodicean church, 'You are neither cold nor hot. I wish you were either one or the other!' (Rev 3:15). So don't let's turn down our church thermostats to a luke-warm temperature—let's turn up the heat by taking these gifts seriously in spite of the extremes some have carried them to. They should never be exercised with brashness, commercialism or sentimentality, but with love, care and sensitivity. Only then can they make a dynamic impact on believers and non-Christians alike.

The gift of faith and the working of miracles

'Is anything too hard for the Lord?' (Gen 18:14)

In Ephesians 3:20 (RSV) Paul cannot find enough words to express what God can do. The apostle has in mind what we ask, but there's more—what 'we ask or think', more again—'all that we ask or think'; more still—'more abundantly than all that we ask or think'. Finally Paul settles for 'far more abundantly than all that we ask or think'. But he emphasizes that it is 'by the power at work within us'.

Since nothing is too hard for the Lord there is no disease that cannot be cured if the correct keys are found and applied. At least one healing evangelist holds an annual service for 'incurables', with tremendous consequences. I am in no way denigrating the excellent work done by hospices in helping people to die with dignity, but I have found in both Scripture and experience countless acts of a miracle-working God.

The gift of working miracles isn't magic but the ability to do things which cannot be done purely through natural means. 400 years ago, if the inhabitants of Birmingham had been told they could see from there what was happening in London they would have denounced this as witchcraft or lunacy or considered it to be a miracle, but now it can easily be achieved through means of television. Similarly, some things which now appear miraculous to us may be taken for granted by our descendants in a 100 years' time. However, God enables some people to do things far beyond the achievements of their own century.

Miracles are among the signs and wonders which confirm the truth of God's work (Mk 16:20). They are signs of his power and works which cause people to wonder at what he has done. When Jesus raised to life the widow of Nain's son the crowd 'were all filled with awe and praised God' (Lk 7:14–16).

Today when Jesus begins to move in miraculous ways the church doesn't always know where to put him. The best thing to do is move with him—to become involved in what he is doing and be ready for him to do it through us.

When miracles happen we don't need to exaggerate them, and when they are explained away we don't need to defend the Lord—he can defend himself. Nor do we need to cheapen them—a small miracle is still a gift of God.

When a schoolteacher had been off work four months with back trouble, Chris and I laid hands on her and she was able to return to school almost immediately. One of her pupils on arriving home that night said, 'Mum, have you heard about the miracle?'

But the gift of working miracles is usually applied to instant healings and unusual happenings. It is always for the benefit of others as Jesus showed. He didn't only use this gift when he was asked to help—he saw the widow of Nain crying and was moved to act knowing that she would appreciate it (Lk 7:13). In a similar way Elisha caused an axe-head to float simply because the man who had dropped it would otherwise have got into trouble for losing it (2 Kings 6:5–7).

Sometimes Christians exclaim, 'We could do with a big miracle, then perhaps people would believe!' But that doesn't necessarily follow—'They will not be convinced even if someone rises from the dead' (Lk 16:31). God's ways are not always our ways (Is 55:9), so our chief motive in working miracles should be to please him whatever happens (1 Cor 10:31). He won't normally expect you to work big miracles before attempting smaller ones, but if you ask for the gift don't be surprised if he puts you into a situation where a miracle is needed.

'SIGNS AND WONDERS AMONG THE PEOPLE' (Acts 5:12)

One kind of miracle is that of multiplication. Just as Jesus fed 5,000 people with five loaves and two fish (Jn 6:1–14), he sometimes makes a little food go a long way. He can do the same with a little money, a little petrol, or a little substance. I read of one brother who with a scant quarter-gallon of paint covered all the walls of his dining room and entrance hall. But that sort of thing only usually happens when Christians are prepared to part with the little they have and trust God to multiply it.

Another type of miracle is that of re-creation—when

the Lord creates new parts for people's bodies. While most healing prayer is for restoration of health or prevention of sickness, sometimes Christians are led to trust for re-creation of bodily organs. Jesus is well able to do this:

> What a spectacle it was! Those who hadn't been able to say a word before were talking excitedly, and those with missing arms and legs had new ones; the crippled were walking and jumping around, and those who had been blind were gazing about them! The crowds just marvelled, and praised the God of Israel (Mt 15:31, The Living Bible).

One example of re-creation today is when the Lord fills people's teeth. A friend of ours was examined by a dentist and told she needed some fillings, but when she kept her appointment for this she was told the dentist was too busy and was asked to come back later. In the meantime she attended a prayer meeting. Then when she did see the dentist he remarked, 'That's funny, your teeth are already filled.'

But the greatest miracle is that of transformation—the miracle of the changed life. An English trader once travelled through what had been cannibal country and he came across a native reading a Bible. 'That book's out of date in my country,' said the trader.

'If it was out of date in my country,' said the native pointing to his mouth, 'you'd have been down there long ago.'

'STAND UP ON YOUR FEET!' (Acts 14:10)

We saw in chapter 5 that the gift of faith is an inrush of faith for a particular occasion and is frequently necessary before instant healings and miracles. We also saw that when the gift is in operation the Christian concerned has no doubt that God is going to do what he is commanding in Jesus' name, and often that he is going to do it then. It is frequently accompanied by a command prayer, as when

Jesus at Nain touched the coffin and said, 'Young man, I say to you, get up!' (Lk 7:14).

The Christian manifesting the gift of faith doesn't ask how, he just knows God will. At that point he is supernaturally emptied of all doubt. No one is like that all the time or we would soon empty the hospitals. But the value of the gift of faith in healing is incalculable. One lady told me she hadn't been able to walk for eight years without her crutch. But I knew that if she stepped out she would, so I encouraged her—and she did.

Many Christians believe God can work miracles but only through great men and women. Yet even Elijah was 'a man just like us'. With gifts of faith he asked God to stop the rain then start it again (Jas 5:17–18), and he called down fire from heaven (1 Kings 18:36–38). God can use ordinary people to do extraordinary acts, and there is no reason why he cannot do through us the sort of things he did through Elijah if we make ourselves available to him.

In some situations a miracle is the only hope for healing and it's right to pray for one. But it may only happen when we step out in faith and obey the Lord on one particular point. The Red Sea waters divided only when Moses stretched out his rod (Ex 14:21). The widow helped by Elisha received a constant supply of oil only after she collected plenty of empty jars from her neighbours (2 Kings 4:1–7). The Lystra cripple was healed only when he obeyed Paul's exhortation to stand up (Acts 14:10).

One reason why miracles happened so frequently in the Indonesian revival was that the Christians involved didn't generally question the possibilities. Like little children they took God at his word (Mt 18:2–3). They read in the Bible that Christ and his disciples worked miracles. They also read that Jesus is the same today (Heb 13:8). So they took it for granted that he would do signs and wonders through them—and he did.

If we spend hours talking about these things our ministry may prove cold and ineffective. If we expect them to happen and get involved when they do, we will be turning on the heat for Jesus.

Gifts and ministries of healing

WHAT GIFTS OF HEALING INVOLVE

A charismatic gift of healing is a supernatural ability to bring Jesus' healing on a specific occasion to a particular person. This is the only gift Paul puts in the plural (1 Cor 12:9), no doubt because there is such a great variety of healing gifts. They are different from natural healing abilities latent in people who are not necessarily Christians, and from psychic healing gifts. Believers who feel they have these other gifts should offer them to the Lord to be channelled for his glory.

Some Christians will manifest spiritual healing gifts more than others, but any believer can be God's channel for them on occasions. However, the gift is not primarily for the channel but for the sick person, and in turn it may benefit others he comes into contact with.

Charismatic healing gifts operate as God determines (1 Cor 12:11). Quite often the Lord wishes to heal through a particular Christian. If you sense he desires to do this through you, you can explain this to the sick person and be led by the Spirit.

Some people are only interested in getting their bodies healed, so we may need to explain that they have other deeper needs, and the purpose of healing gifts is also to open the way for wholeness. Of the ten lepers who came to Jesus nine were cleansed and healed but only one was made completely whole—the one who returned to thank him (Lk 17:11–19). However dramatic a healing may be, what Chris and I desire more than anything is for the person who has received it to go away with the healer, not just the healing; with the giver, not just the gift.

How gifts of healing differ

God bestows a variety of healing gifts so that different Christians can use them in different contexts like nursing, counselling, social work, evangelism, deliverance ministry, and many other areas. High success in a particular context may mean a believer has a particular ministry for that area. If every Christian used all the gifts available to him we would be able to tell the world what Jesus told John the Baptist, 'The blind receive sight, the lame walk, those who have leprosy are cured, the deaf hear, the dead are raised, and the good news is preached to the poor' (Lk 7:22).

A couple were leaving church one evening when someone asked them for healing ministry. Another Sunday someone else asked them for the same thing. In each case the request came without warning, it concerned knee trouble, and the afflicted person was healed through the couple's prayer. This couple soon concluded that the Lord was using them in a ministry to knees. A girl, meanwhile, found she had a ministry to migraines. Then there was a young man with a ministry to backs, who frequently witnessed people's backs getting healed as he laid hands on their feet and the shorter of their two legs grew to the size of the other. Since back trouble is so common, he literally had his hands full. But he was proving the truth of Psalm 146:8 which can be rendered 'He straightens the backs of those that are bent.'

Gifts of healing are used in a variety of service. With the advent of cable television to our country comes the daunting possibility of viewing American healing evangelists any hour of the day or night. Some of these have a very different approach from British ones. Some Christian healers major on the word of knowledge in their ministries, some on the communion, some on anointing with oil, some, like Chris and I, on the laying-on-of-hands. We

need to take the best from any ministry and allow for
different kinds of service, remembering it's done to the
same Lord (1 Cor 12:5).

People with healing gifts use a variety of methods. God
isn't limited to sacramental or charismatic, high church or
low, traditional churches or new ones. If we are open to
the Spirit in our healing ministries he will use us in new
ways besides those we are already experienced in. Chris
has never been trained in massage, but one day she found
herself giving a skilful massage to a lady's back. The
woman remarked on the warmth and comfort this form of
treatment was bringing her. The more we grow in healing
gifts the more the Lord leads us into newer and more
exciting dimensions of ministry.

WHAT GIFTS OF HEALING DEMAND

'How do I know if I have a gift of healing?' Usually when
someone asks this question he means a ministry of healing, for no one has a healing gift except during the short
time it's being channelled through him. It's another gift
which you often only know afterwards that you've exercised.

No Christian has any right to set himself up as a healer.
Believers with healing ministries usually started simply by
obeying Jesus' command to heal the sick whenever they
had opportunity (Lk 10:9). The way they and others knew
they had manifested healing gifts or had healing ministries
was when people were constantly healed through their
prayers.

Occasionally at the close of a meeting someone has
approached Chris or me and said, 'While you were laying
hands on people I had a tingling in my hands. Do you
think the Lord is calling me to a healing ministry?'

We have then replied, 'Hold on. It may be the first sign,
but there's a lot more to it than that.' We go on to remind
the person of all the suffering we went through before our

ministry came to fruition, as described in *It Hurts to Heal*. Not everyone has the same sort of preparation, but much confirmation is required before a Christian assumes he has a healing ministry.

However, when a Christian lady at Barking spoke of a tingling in her hands she added that she had experienced this every time she had seen the laying-on-of-hands during the previous ten years. We encouraged her to launch out into ministry at the earliest opportunity as the Lord definitely seemed to be saying something to her.

But just how do you launch into a ministry of healing? Again, the principle 'every case is different' applies. If you listen to the Lord as you pray with the sick and obey him at each stage you may find such a ministry just develops. But for a public healing ministry it's important not only that you know the Lord's call but that other Christians recognize it too. So if you feel the Lord is calling you to a public healing ministry the next step may be to approach your pastor.

I was thrown in at the deep end when Trevor Dearing felt the Lord was calling me to such a ministry and invited me to assist him at a healing service in his church. Chris, meanwhile, was three times shown by the Lord that he would use her hands to bless millions. When this was confirmed I encouraged her to assist me in my own parish church and people quickly discovered that her ministry was genuine.

How can we prepare for a work of healing? Jesus said, 'To whom much is given, of him will much be required' (Lk 12:48 RSV). As we're living in such exciting days and as we're privileged to see so much happening we have an immense responsibility to serve the Lord in our different areas of ministry whatever the cost. We may have to make time to acquire training in the healing ministry. The Lord can use the untrained but he won't do much with those who are not prepared to learn. There's no preparation of the sick in the Gospels but there's plenty of preparation of the ministers of healing.

We will also need to be ready to cope with the results, good and bad. Amazingly some Christians won't accept that people have been healed through prayer, even when the evidence is right under their noses. One lady cured of leg trouble found her Christian friends just couldn't cope with her healing. 'They'd rather I was back on crutches!' she exclaimed. We will have to be prepared never to be 'off duty'. Once people know you have a ministry of healing you may be called upon anywhere to help those in need. A friend of ours found herself ministering Jesus' touch in a ladies' cloakroom.

But the benefits far outweigh the difficulties, the rewards far surpass the effort, the job-satisfaction is high and the long-term consequences immeasurable. There is a tremendous need for wholehearted believers who will say to the sick and troubled, 'What I have I give you' (Acts 3:6). There are millions of desperate, captive, oppressed and afflicted people who are waiting for you and me to turn on the heat. Dare we disappoint them?

Suggested reading: Luke 7:11–23.

Key 5

POWER: THE KEY TO SPIRITUAL IGNITION

15

Christians Entrusted with Dynamite

About thirty ministers and their wives had gathered at Mabledon Conference Centre near Tonbridge to hear Chris and me sharing about our healing ministry. I had just finished outlining the six keys to healing when one of the ministers declared, 'My church has recently been challenged by Jesus' words to the Sadducees, "You are in error because you do not know the Scriptures or the power of God" (Mt 22:29). Most of the keys are in evidence in my church but it's a release of power we're lacking.'

This is the experience of so many fellowships, and one reason why the Christian church has often failed to heal is because it has neglected the power. Yet that power is at our fingertips and it's mightier than nuclear energy. It's the same power that brought this universe into being and brought Jesus back from the dead. Christians are the most powerful people in the world.

Jesus promised his disciples, 'You will receive power when the Holy Spirit comes on you' (Acts 1:8). The Greek word used for power here and in many other places is *dunamis* from which we get our word dynamite. It indicates might and ability. But whereas dynamite is used for destructive purposes, the power of the Holy Spirit is especially given for the constructive work of evangelism and healing.

Jesus took a risk by entrusting Christians with spiritual dynamite, because dynamite is always dangerous. Some believers have been playing with fire instead of praying with fire, and some have let the power go to their heads. But where the dynamite has been wisely used, it's often been the key that has unlocked the door to healing.

Why do we require the dynamite?

CHRISTIANS ARE RESTRICTED WITHOUT IT

There was once a fire at a village church. Who should turn out to fight the blaze with the other locals but Mr Smith the village atheist. The Vicar seized his opportunity and remarked, 'This is the first time I've seen you in my church, Mr Smith,' to which the atheist replied, 'This is the first time I've seen your church on fire.' Thank God that many churches are now being set on fire by the dynamite of God the Holy Spirit! Others, however, present the facts and the faith in an orderly way but need the fire to ignite them.

Many Christians have experienced their Good Friday and Easter Day—they have died to sin and risen with Christ to newness of life (Rom 6:11)—but they have halted somewhere between Calvary and Pentecost. Others have gone on to experience their Ascension Day and Whit Sunday—they have made Jesus king of their lives and received a definite outpouring of the Holy Spirit's power (Acts 2:33).

In the healing ministry we become channels of tremendous power. But the tap cannot turn itself on—as a channel it's dependent on someone outside it to start the flow.

Similarly, we are dependent on the power of God. 'Why do you stare at us,' asked Peter, 'as if by our own power or godliness we had made this man walk?' (Acts 3:12). We shouldn't make our unworthiness as channels an excuse for holding back. A watering-can is not very attractive to look at but it can be a very effective channel. Paul was aware of how Christians sometimes feel inadequate when he wrote, 'We have this treasure in jars of clay to show that this all-surpassing power is from God and not from us' (2 Cor 4:7).

HEALING IS RESTRICTED WITHOUT IT

At one point in his Gospel Doctor Luke comments, 'The power of the Lord was present for him [Jesus] to heal the sick' (Lk 5:17). This suggests that sometimes the power was not present in the sense of being released. Today the power is present in every believer, for every true Christian has the Holy Spirit (Rom 8:9). But it is not always released, and this can prove an inhibiting factor in healing. The radio provides a useful illustration. The potential is always within it, but unless it's switched on and the power flows through it, no programme can be received.

When I first read Kathryn Kuhlman's books about folk who had been healed through her ministry of the word of knowledge in America I was puzzled. Each testimony described how a sick person had usually been ministered to at least once elsewhere but had shown little obvious improvement, yet once he attended her meeting he experienced a remarkable recovery. 'Why was this?' I pondered.

I concluded it wasn't just because Kathryn was an exceptionally gifted lady. There must have been something about the atmosphere in her meetings that made a difference. Atmosphere is always important in healing, whether in church, home or hospital, and if the atmosphere is a powerful one—in the sense that healing energy is being freely released in powerful ways—we are more likely to see results.

At one of our own meetings the Lord promised, 'Volcanoes will erupt soon around you, and many will feel the effects.' Two years later we noticed this coming to pass in churches represented at that meeting. Mighty manifestations of the Spirit were in evidence, and Chris and I were able to visit some churches that only twelve months previously had been unprepared for a powerful healing ministry.

How do we receive the dynamite?

A CONSCIOUS EXPERIENCE OF THE SPIRIT

Sometimes people find healing at the same time as they are filled with the Holy Spirit, like blind Saul of Tarsus at Straight Street in Damascus (Acts 9:17–18). Probably the majority of Christians now ministering healing have been baptized in the Spirit like the church on the Day of Pentecost (Acts 1:5). They were all filled (Acts 2:4), but what seemed like tongues of fire rested on each of them (Acts 2:3). So we can expect the Lord to release his power among whole fellowships, but this process often begins as individual Christians experience a renewal in their personal lives and then bring the fruits of this into their congregations.

The baptism in the Holy Spirit is available to every believer (Acts 2:38–39). It's a free gift from Jesus, and some Christians find it just happens to them as they are washing the dishes or mowing the lawn. But being filled with the Spirit is sometimes compared with drinking (1 Cor 12:13). Drinking is a conscious act, and it is as we appropriate what we ask for that we find we have received it. Dr Torrey noted that he had met many people who were born again and didn't realize it, whereas he had never met anyone who was baptized in the Spirit without knowing it—

even if it was called by some other name.

When we seek this release of power it should be for God's glory and on his terms. But if a person is born again, renounces any occult involvement, is thirsty for the Lord, asks to be filled, believes the Lord is doing it and speaks out trusting the Holy Spirit to give him the words, there is no reason normally why such a person shouldn't receive and know it. If he doesn't, it's a matter of trusting and persevering until he does.

A CONTINUOUS OVERFLOW OF THE SPIRIT

We know when a vessel is really filled when it overflows. Healing power is also released as Christians overflow.

I was once preparing a girl for confirmation and I explained how we need to be filled with the Spirit so that we have more power to witness for Christ (Acts 1:8). 'Oh, I don't need that!' she exclaimed. 'I already witness at school.'

'But can you say like Peter and John,' I enquired, 'We cannot help speaking about what we have seen and heard?' (Acts 4:20). The girl admitted she couldn't, and added, 'Perhaps I do need this power after all.'

When we're filled to overflowing we sometimes find ourselves saying and doing things we would never dream of planning to do. Consequently healing flows more freely and miracles occur more frequently.

How do we renew the dynamite?

KEEP GETTING FILLED

When Paul told the Ephesians, 'Be filled with the Spirit' (Eph 5:18), he meant 'keep coming back to get filled.' When D. L. Moody was asked why he needed so many fillings of the Holy Spirit he replied, 'I leak.'

After a lot of use, clothing wears out and needs to be

renewed. In extreme heat liquids dry up and need to be renewed. Under certain circumstances batteries go flat and need to be recharged. Now the overflow of the Spirit is automatic but the filling is not. We have already seen that New Testament Christians knew when they were filled and always opened their mouths as a result. So every time I ask the Lord to refill me with his power I immediately open my mouth and speak to him or for him. That way I'm prepared for healing ministry.

Particular occasions when we need to be filled again are before opportunities to speak or minister for the Lord, before difficult tasks, and at the beginning of each day. Sometimes we may wish to be refilled through receiving ourselves the ministry of laying-on-of-hands and so be equipped through a fresh touch from the Lord. This particularly applies when we have been away from him, when we're spiritually dry, and when we're conscious that barriers in our lives are blocking the flow of his healing power through us.

SET JESUS FREE

The flow of the Holy Spirit can be continuous all the time it's not blocked. But sometimes Christians are like a river in Africa which makes its way towards the sea and never gets there. When we're aware of things in our lives which grieve the Holy Spirit (Eph 4:30) we'll want to be emptied of them so that we can be clearer channels of healing. A certain amount of water may still get through a clogged drainpipe, and it's not true to say God can only use completely pure channels, but we'll be better channels if we're clean throughout and the power of God is flowing freely through our lives.

Every year at the feast of the Passover Pilate the governor 'was in the habit of setting free for the people any one prisoner whom they chose' (Mt 27:15 Amplified Version). But when he had the opportunity to release Jesus he kept him bound. We too can keep Jesus bound by keeping his power locked up inside us, but, if we get into the habit of setting him free to do what he wants, his healing power will flow through us with no restrictions.

This applies not only to individuals but also to churches. Though many are being set alight, the fire is sometimes allowed to spread no further. Church leaders sometimes quench the Holy Spirit (1 Thess 5:19) because they are frightened things will get out of control. Yet only as we allow Jesus to work powerfully will we see not only renewal but revival, not only fellowships coming alive but whole communities transformed as well.

How do we release the dynamite?

How can we see more healing power released in our churches?

OPEN YOUR MOUTH

'Be filled with the Spirit. Speak to one another with psalms, hymns and spiritual songs. Sing and make music in your heart to the Lord, always giving thanks to God the Father for everything in the name of our Lord Jesus Christ' (Eph 5:18–20).

When the Holy Spirit came at Pentecost, prayer turned into praise (Acts 1:14; 2:11), and praise—not just singing and rejoicing but Spirit-filled adoration—releases power. Healing power is also released through united prayer. I used to wonder what difference it made for Christians to pray unitedly rather than individually. Then I realized that the devil can more easily distract or confuse one believer on his own, whereas he is literally frightened when Christians pray together in power.

The word spoken with authority can release healing energy. So can gifts of the Spirit and the powerful gift of tongues. Sometimes when Chris and I don't know the root cause of a person's sickness we pray in tongues and it comes to light. And sometimes when all else has failed we ask the Lord to give us a tongue for the situation. Kevin from Leigh-on-Sea, who attended the first Breath Fellowship residential conference, told me he had suffered from shoulder pain for some time.

'I kept receiving ministry,' Kevin explained, 'but the pain didn't go. So I asked the Lord to give me the appropriate tongue for the problem. I then found myself praying in a language I'd never used before. The pain went instantly, and it's never come back since.'

As individuals are released in the Spirit and pray regularly in tongues they can become charged up like human dynamos, so that when they come together and open their mouths the effects can be dynamic and the Lord stretches out his hand to heal (Acts 4:30).

OPEN YOUR HANDS

Something always happens when Christians lay hands on people in Jesus' name. His touch has still its ancient power, and the power of touch is added to the power of prayer. When one lady discovered this she said to Chris and me, 'I wish I could gather my sick friends and relatives in this room—then you could touch them all.'

Reflexologists believe that by massaging people's feet they are releasing healing energy which helps trigger the body's healing system and speed up natural processes of healing. Christians believe something similar happens through touch in Jesus' name, but that God can also add supernatural power and gifts in the process. When a glass reflects the sun's heat onto a piece of paper it can burn a hole in the paper because the power is concentrated in one place. The same sort of thing happens in the laying-on-of-hands as healing energy from God is transmitted through the hands of the channel to the person in need (Mk 5:31). It's like a car with a flat battery being made to go by a car with a well-charged one. In soaking prayer the same thing happens over a long period of time. Healing energy soaks in at the point of contact, such as the neck if we're laying hands on the neck, but other areas of the body or personality may derive benefit in the process.

Healing may be hindered by resistance, tension or negative attitudes in either the sufferer or the person ministering. It may not happen, either, if we use the powerful touch as an excuse for ignoring natural, God-given powers we possess like taking exercise. While laying hands on ourselves may sometimes lead to healing, at other times this can have the effect of 'short-circuiting' the blessing.

What else will result from the dynamite?

A NEW DIMENSION OF LIVING

When believers are baptized in the Spirit they have a new appreciation of the supernatural dimension. When it happened to Chris she had a new awareness of the reality of Jesus, though at first she didn't know how to relate her experience to her ministry. When it happened to me my ministry took on a different approach as I began to expect God to work signs and wonders through me which would point people to Jesus—what John Wimber calls power evangelism (Acts 8:6). I began to understand what it means to be 'aglow with the Spirit' (Rom 12:11 RSV).

This supernatural dimension includes physical manifestations of the Spirit's power. Chris in particular experiences these, as she once prayed that the Lord would make himself real to her in tangible ways. All these manifestations are expressions of the powerful touch of Jesus. Feeling is not the same as filling, but we believe that if the Lord touches our bodies we should yield to what he is doing.

Sometimes Chris's arms fill with power and it literally

hurts her to heal. She has to discharge the energy into the needy person, an experience she has sometimes compared to having a baby. At other times her hands will vibrate as she ministers.

After *It Hurts to Heal* was published, a number of Christians wrote to say how they were so glad they weren't the only ones with such 'strange' manifestations. But, if when the early church prayed the building was shaken (Acts 4:31), we shouldn't be surprised if sometimes the Holy Spirit takes people off their feet or anoints their bodies in tangible ways. He will come upon us in power if we allow him to.

A DIFFERENT LEVEL OF CONSCIOUSNESS

One of the things that can happen when we yield to the Spirit is that we enter temporarily into a different level of consciousness. We're not unconscious but 'resting in the Spirit'. Under certain circumstances our regular beta brainwaves change to alpha ones. This can happen through harmful experimentation with hard drugs or transcendental meditation, but it can also happen during Spirit-filled worship, contemplative meditation on the Lord, and under the ministry of laying-on-of-hands. In particular we often rest in the Spirit after falling under God's power. A number of people fell under this power in the Bible (Acts 9:4; Rev 1:17), and the soldiers fell backwards in the Garden of Gethsemane when Jesus used the powerful name of God, 'I am' (Jn 18:6).

Resting in the Spirit on the floor is now extremely widespread, and seems to be linked less with particular ministers as with powerful atmospheres. It has taken place in great evangelistic crusades and also at Anglican theological colleges where the staff have been laying on hands. We should beware of aiming to fall, but if we resist the power we may miss out on a blessing. God won't force anyone to fall who is tense or resistant, and no minister can make it take place, but it can be a beautiful experience for those who let it happen as a by-product of the ministry. Resting in the Spirit doesn't necessarily mean a person is healed or baptized in the Spirit. It's simply a sign that God's power has been released and Jesus is working in our midst (Mk 16:20).

While on the floor people are usually at their most relaxed, so God may be ministering to them at deeper levels of their subconscious quite apart from the ministry we have given them. Many have been convicted of sin, drawn closer to Jesus, seen visions, or found fresh strength for living, and these blessings have shown in the radiance of their faces as they have returned to their seats afterwards. Falling under the power sometimes occurs when no one is laying hands on people and when those concerned are at a distance from the ministers. Chris and I always point the congregation beyond such experiences to our mighty God, and give him the glory (Heb 2:4).

It can be undignified if people keel over while kneeling, so in our own ministry at meetings we usually ask folk to stand while we lay hands on them, and have catchers on hand to lower them gently to the floor. This is purely for reassurance as no harm has come to people who have fallen without catchers. But these stewards can also look after spectacles, earpieces and crutches while the ministry is proceeding, and be prepared to help people to their feet again when they are eventually ready.

These are just some of the effects of the dynamite Jesus entrusts us with. If we release this power more, we'll not only see more people healed but we'll be writing history. For the Acts of the Apostles ends abruptly at chapter twenty-eight, but you and I can, in one sense, help to write chapter twenty-nine.

Suggested readings: Acts 2:1–21; Ephesians 5:15–21.

16

You Can Use My Name

John Newton was a drunken slave-trader who frequently used Jesus' name as a swear word. But Newton was converted, and later became Rector of Olney. In 1779 he wrote the hymn 'How sweet the name of Jesus sounds in a believer's ear'. 'Jesus' was by then to Newton a precious name, for to a believer 'It soothes his sorrows, heals his wounds', but it was also a powerful name, for 'it drives away his fear'.

The name of Jesus is still a powerful name, not in a superstitious sense but as a means by which God's power is released to save, heal and deliver. Many people when lonely, frightened or in the dark, have whispered that name and known instant peace. One scientist even discovered that more radiation than usual was given off when the name of Jesus was spoken. One day a woman in the grip of evil started walking around a church and tearing up Bibles. 'Stop,' called out the minister, 'in the name of Jesus!' She stopped immediately.

Where the Lord's name is uplifted his presence is felt and his glory is manifested, but also his authority is adhered to. He has given authority to all believers to use that powerful, authoritative name—'In my name they will drive out demons; they will speak in new tongues; they will pick up snakes with their hands; and when they drink deadly poison, it will not hurt them at all; they will place their hands on sick people, and they will get well' (Mk 16:17–18).

When the police knock at a suspect's door and shout, 'Open up in the name of the law!' they have behind them all the authority of the courts. And when we minister to people and invite them to open up their lives in the name of Jesus, we have behind us all the authority of the King of kings.

The authority given us by Jesus and centred in his name is another kind of power which needs to be released for healing. The dynamite can only be used safely if backed up by the right authority, so in this chapter we will look at what it means to have Christ's authority. Let's remember that whatever need we're ministering to, Jesus says to every one of us, 'You can use my name.'

Under authority

The centurion who came to Jesus to ask for healing for his sick slave said, 'I myself am a man under authority' (Mt 8:9). Although he had a hundred soldiers under him he could only give orders because he was able to take them. Christians can only expect to take authority over sickness and evil if they are prepared to submit—to the Lord, the Bible, and those in the church they are responsible to. Three homely pictures may help to illustrate this.

A PAIR OF SCALES

Like so many aspects of the healing ministry, the exercise of authority can sometimes be 'weighed on the scales and found wanting' (Dan 5:27), for it can be unbalanced at one end or the other. At one extreme, authority can be exercised in such a way that the people given commands are deprived of their freedom to be themselves. This happens when Christians seek power without obeying the Lord and so impose themselves and their personalities upon people.

At the other extreme, everyone does what is 'right in his own eyes' (Judg 21:25 AV) and recognizes no authority over him. Yet one consequence that should result from being filled with the Spirit is the ability to 'submit to one another out of reverence for Christ' (Eph 5:21). This submission cannot be forcibly imposed by church law but will often result from Christians seeing Jesus in other believers. Although there are occasions when we have to say, 'We must obey God rather than men!' (Acts 5:29), our authority in healing will have little effect unless we are prepared to be people under authority.

The balance Jesus is looking for in the exercise of authority lies somewhere between these two extremes. It means exercising authority while making room for true freedom (2 Cor 3:17).

A PIECE OF SANDWICH

Cut it through the centre and you find the filling, with one layer of bread above it and another layer below it. Every Christian ministering healing is like the filling in that sandwich. We are each responsible to those above us and also to those who look up to us for direction. Jesus took orders from God; he would say and do nothing unless his Father wanted it (Jn 5:30; 8:28). He could give orders to his disciples—'As the Father has sent me, I am sending you' (Jn 20:21). But when he exercised his authority it was with the humility of a servant, and he said, 'I, your Lord and Teacher, have washed your feet, you also should wash one another's feet' (Jn 13:14).

Those who exercise particular authority in the church need to have been clearly called by God and have their authority recognized by the church. Such authority is not derived from their institutional position or personal magnetism but from God. Those who minister healing need to be more like Jesus—listening to the Father so that they are ready to act on his behalf.

A PERSON'S SIGNATURE

When the leper said to Jesus, 'If you are willing, you can make me clean' (Mt 8:2), Jesus replied, 'I am willing . . . be clean!' (Mt 8:3). The Lord's 'I will' was like the signature of a doctor on a document authorizing treatment.

We Christians can say, 'I will,' when people ask us to minister to them, and in Jesus' name we can authorize treatment. But we're only entitled to do this if we first say, 'I will' to him.

During an election we vote people into power and authority by putting crosses, a form of signature, against their names. Similarly, we can give authority in our daily lives to either Jesus or Satan. Every thought or act of fear gives the enemy a little power over us, while every thought or act of faith gives the Lord more power over us.

Taking authority

Jesus derived his authority from the Father, we derive ours from Jesus. His authority was not like that of the scribes—wishy-washy or cold-hearted (Mt 7:29)—but positive yet tender. We can command healing and blessing in his name with the same firmness and gentleness.

COMMANDING HEALING AND BLESSING

Peter used a command prayer with the lame man at the Beautiful Gate—'In the name of Jesus Christ of Nazareth, walk' (Acts 3:6). He then took him by the right hand and lifted him up (Acts 3:7). In the Middle East the left hand is regarded as the hand of filth while the right hand is the hand of power. Jesus is seated at the right hand of God

(Mk 16:19) where all authority has been given to him (Mt 28:18). So as we command healing in Jesus' name and help the sick to their feet we see the King of kings go into action. We also have his authority to proclaim forgiveness of sins and deliverance from evil.

COMING AGAINST OUR ENEMIES

'For our struggle is not against flesh and blood, but against . . . the spiritual forces of evil in the heavenly realms' (Eph 6:12). When evil forces come against us, in whatever shape or form, we can come against them with the authority of Christ.

We can come against them with resistance. James writes, 'Resist the devil, and he will flee from you' (Jas 5:7). God has put all things under Jesus' feet (Eph 1:22) and we are seated with him in heavenly places (Eph 2:6). Therefore our enemies are under our feet too, and, as Charles Wesley reminds us, we can 'tread all the powers of darkness down'.

The simplest form of deliverance, one possible for any believer, is letting go. Some difficulties are too big for us to overcome through our own prayers, but others can be overcome as we simply claim the victory Jesus has won for us (1 Cor 15:57) and in his name resist the devil, recognizing that he is the source of the fear, the misunderstanding, or whatever the problem may be.

However, when Jesus said believers would be safe if they picked up snakes (Mk 16:18), he didn't mean (as some sects in America believe) that Christians will be safe if they deliberately do this. That's like saying I'll be protected if I deliberately walk under a bus. But if we're walking in the Lord's will and clothed in his armour (Eph 6:11), we'll be safe even if all we can do is stand firm (Eph 6:14).

When Jesus was tempted he resisted the devil by using the sword of the Spirit, the word of God (Eph 6:17). Each time he was attacked he answered, 'It is written' (Lk 4:4, 8, 10). If we get to know our Bibles we shall be ready to resist, and the promise is that the devil will run away fast.

There are times, however, when we're not only to defend ourselves but also to attack the Enemy, and the simplest form of attack is rebuking. Jesus rebuked demons (Mt 17:18), sicknesses (Lk 4:39) and other forms of evil. We can come against any barriers Satan puts in our way, and when we do we will see Jesus' victory in action.

There are also times when we're to leave the rebuking to God, as did the archangel Michael when disputing about the body of Moses (Jude 9). But the context there is not one of healing, and we seldom come face to face with the devil himself as Michael did—most of the time we're dealing with his agents. So we cannot use this reference as an excuse for not rebuking evil powers—that's exactly what Satan would like us to do. Most of the time it's up to us to rebuke the enemy with the authority Christ has given us.

'Affliction go, in Jesus' name!' is one rebuking prayer which has sometimes unlocked the door to instant healing, especially of conditions like deafness, hernias, trapped nerves and back trouble. There's no need always to shout when rebuking, though if we're calling upon the Enemy to surrender we don't do it in a whisper.

A lady called Glenys had a husband who constantly beat and ill-treated her. But she began to see his attacks as motivated by the devil, so each time he went for her she would cry, 'I rebuke you, evil spirit, in the name of Jesus!' Instantly on each occasion the man either turned deathly pale or was thrown back across the room by the mighty power of God.

Jesus has also given authority to Christians to restrict evil powers. He promised, 'Whatever you bind on earth will be bound in heaven' (Mt 18:18). When we address specific evil forces and say, 'We bind you in the name of

Jesus,' this has the effect of leaving them bound and gagged so that they are unable to harm anyone present, just as when God shut the mouths of the lions that would have devoured Daniel (Dan 6:22).

Sometimes people become frightened when they see God's power manifested. This may be because they are witnessing something new to them, and their particular backgrounds may not have prepared them for such manifestations. In most cases their fears can be overcome through caring, explanation and persistence. But the reason some people react is because evil spirits have a hold upon them and are terrified by the power of God.

When such folk scream out or react in other demonstrative ways it's often right to bind the evil spirits concerned, and if exorcism is to follow it's always wise to do so. Jesus asked, 'How can anyone enter a strong man's house and carry off his possessions unless he first ties up the strong man?' (Mt 12:29).

The same applies when we are bothered by particular evil forces. At a midweek meeting in a Baptist chapel a man would regularly get up, wander around, and distract people from the worship. Roy, the minister, recognized this as the enemy's work, so each week before the meeting he would bind all evil powers from those who attended it. From then on the difficult man gave no further trouble, until one day Roy and his wife Priscilla went on holiday. That week no one else thought of binding Satan from the meeting and the man was soon up to his old tricks again.

Jesus also gave believers the authority to release people from evil and harmful things. He promised, 'Whatever you loose on earth will be loosed in heaven' (Mt 18:18). This is the most common form of deliverance, and something else which any believer has authority to do under the Holy Spirit's leading. However, as some problems sometimes prove to be more complicated than envisaged, it's again usually best for inexperienced Christians to let others take the lead.

We have seen that when a problem is small it may be overcome through our own personal prayers as it's like a piece of string which can easily be snapped. But when a problem is like a big chain around us we may need someone else to use the appropriate key to unlock the chain in Jesus' name. As the sword of the Spirit can cut through chains, Christians can speak God's word to people who are bound to harmful things and say, 'We cut you free in the name of Jesus.' As one woman was set free in this way from bondage to her mother, her sister, who was miles away, simultaneously shook from head to foot. The same sort of powerful effects have resulted when curses put on people by satanists or black witches have been broken by the authority of Christ.

In a later chapter we'll look more closely at what it means to be loosed from bondages. But there are two other forms of deliverance Jesus has given the church authority to do—sending off and casting out. Fearful, inexperienced and untrained Christians should never take a lead in either of these, which include sending evil forces away from places they are haunting or people they are oppressing, and driving out demons from people they are inhabiting and possessing. But once again the victory is assured for those who are led by the Spirit.

CASTING OUT EVIL SPIRITS

Believers who cast out demons find it an exhilarating but costly experience. Sometimes it means spending several days in prayer and fasting (Mk 9:29 AV), and Satan's agents get to know those they are dealing with face to face (Acts 19:15). We may be subject to seasons of attack from them, especially before or after particular projects for the Lord.

But when oppressed or battered we can claim promises like Isaiah 59:17 (AV)—'When the enemy shall come in like a flood, the Spirit of the Lord shall lift up a standard against him.' If we go into battle with praise we will witness the victory—'As they began to sing and praise, the Lord set ambushes against the men . . . who were invading Judah, and they were defeated' (2 Chron 20:22).

It's frequently necessary to discern the cause of demon-possession before we can begin casting out demons. The demonized people who need deliverance may not be aware of the cause when they first come into contact with us, but we have already seen how we can discern where Satan has a hold.

In some cases this is only too clear. Angela was sent by a witches' coven to pray against a Christian service, but the Lord spoke to her and she was converted. She had, however, sold her soul to Satan, writing this in blood. So when we came against a demon in her it cried, 'She's mine!'—and it took six men to hold Angela down as her arms were filled with superhuman strength. But after she had undone her pact with Satan and put in writing that she had given her life to Christ, Angela was set free over a period from each of the demons that possessed her, one by one. She was eventually baptized, and cared for by students at a theological college.

In cases of multiple possession we get to know when we are dealing with some demons that are stronger than others. Quite often there are two 'bodyguards', perhaps mocking spirits that cause the person to giggle or jeer when taken over. Then may follow the stronger demon which has often come through connection with the occult.

At a service near Worthing a possessed girl looked at me with hatred in her eyes as I bent over her. She was delivered in Jesus' name, but the next day told me she had wanted to kill me. I was unafraid, however, remembering again that Jesus' power is stronger than that of hatred or murder. But some evil spirits project less obvious manifestations. If a person becomes obsessed with resentment a

demon may attach itself to that person and when exposed
to God's power its only manifestation may be a possible
sneer in the face. When the spirit leaves, it likewise does
so less obviously. But the fact of the deliverance should
come clear in time as the person who has had the spirit of
resentment exhibits instead an attitude of love and forgiveness.

Casting out demons involves directly challenging them.
Some Christians prefer not to lay hands on a person while
he is taken over by powers of darkness, and while the
touch is ministered for healing it's usually the word for
deliverance. Jesus 'drove out the spirits with a word' (Mt
8:16). Note that he didn't lead them out but drove them
out. There's no point in saying, 'Please will you come
out?' A command prayer of authority is required as the
demon is challenged to leave in Jesus' name (Acts 16:18).

Having claimed the protection of Christ's blood and
bound the spirit, we don't then start arguing with it. When
Winston Churchill was once asked what his answer was to
a message sent him by Hitler, he growled, 'I cannot reply
to someone with whom I am not on speaking terms.' And
when we're in the forefront of the battle we don't send
telegrams to the enemy.

Evil spirits must be told to go, even when they are not
inhabiting a person's body, and if Jesus' name is used they
have to bow to his authority. When one man came against
a spirit of infirmity, the child involved stopped in mid-
scream. Some demons leave instantly when ordered to,
like the one that mocked Jesus in the synagogue (Lk
4:35). Others only depart after a struggle, like Legion in
the demoniac among the tombs (Mk 5:6–13). But all must
leave eventually if commanded to in Jesus' name and if
those people they have holds on have renounced them.

It's wisest also to tell the spirits where to go, just as
Jesus caused Legion to go into a herd of pigs (Mk 5:11–
13). Chris and I always say to a demon, 'Go to where

Jesus sends you!'—and eventually it does. But this challenge cannot easily be given at a distance, or over the telephone. Direct ministry is necessary if actual possession is involved, not only because the person concerned also needs building up but because evil spirits can usually only understand what we say to them aloud. Although Satan has power to drop thoughts into our minds, and although his agents pick up a certain amount of supernatural knowledge from him as we can from the Lord, they cannot automatically read our thoughts and they need to hear the command.

When someone has been released from demon-possession he is in need of care. While in the grip of the Enemy that person shouldn't be seen as evil but invaded by a hostile force. Nevertheless, since that person wittingly or unwittingly invited it in by an act of his will, it will only depart if by an act of will it is renounced along with the sin that originally attracted it to gain hold. An ounce of confession is worth a ton of exorcism, and Chris and I have discovered that the more the needy person co-operates in the deliverance the more easily the demon leaves.

Afterwards it's our responsibility to see that the released captive is given care and fellowship and that he keeps close to the Lord and away from those activities which might invite other evil forces in by the back door to take the place of those demons who have left by the front door (Mt 12:43–45). Then, as long as all concerned continue to claim the Lord's protection, there's nothing to fear.

Suggested reading: Matthew 8:1–17.

17

Built-in Central Heating

The manufacturers of a well-known brand of instant porridge advertised their product as 'central heating for kids'. Children were seen enjoying the porridge, then setting off into a cold day each completely surrounded by a haze of light.

This chapter is about built-in central heating for Christians. It concerns another aspect of power for healing which is sometimes overlooked—the anointing of the Holy Spirit. When Jesus first proclaimed the healing he had come to bring he announced in the words of Isaiah, 'The Spirit of the Lord is on me, because he has anointed me' (Lk 4:18; cf. Is 61:1).

What the anointing means

IT'S A TRADEMARK

Anointing has different meanings but we're especially thinking of it here as an obvious outpouring of the Holy Spirit in power upon a Christian or group of believers. It's normally a conscious experience, for it can be compared with the pouring of oil on a person's head, and such a

199

person would be aware of that unless he was asleep, unconscious or dead. Others present would also be aware of what was happening, and in the same way the anointing is a spiritual 'trademark' which may be noticed by other people. When the Spirit comes upon us it should be obvious, and when the anointing is missing that should be evident too.

It's difficult to appreciate exactly what's involved in anointing unless you have experienced it yourself, for it's a mysterious and sovereign work of God. However, it's definitely not just an emotional experience but a spiritual one. A healing service doesn't have to be emotional or noisy to have the anointing upon it. Nor is unction the same as earnestness. An anointed Christian will be earnest but you can be earnest without the anointing.

Sometimes I'm tired or tense while ministering and I know the anointing is not upon me. Thank God he can still bless many present in spite of me. But my ministry on such occasions doesn't have the same power (1 Cor 2:4-5). When the anointing isn't there I cannot force it to come. Sometimes we leaders try to organize the Spirit in our meetings instead of moving under his anointing. But our ministry will be most effective if, when we come to lay on hands, we pray the prayer of faith (Jas 5:15), then move out of the way and let the Lord do what he desires.

IT'S TANGIBLE

Jesus can not only touch our bodies through the laying-on-of-hands, he can anoint us anywhere, any time. My wife and I were once viewing some articles in a furniture shop when the Lord's anointing came upon Chris and she was bathed in his power. And while we're not to rely on feelings, we may be encouraged by the feel of the Lord's touch upon any part of our bodies.

A lady in one of our London meetings, however, wasn't used to this when she felt a movement upon her stomach (she had stomach trouble). Later she told Chris and me, 'I went outside to walk it off.'

'You don't walk off the Spirit,' we laughed, 'you walk in him!' (Gal 5:25).

Not only can the anointing be felt, it can sometimes be seen. Some Christians have seen lights around us and others, just like those in the porridge advertisement. Again, this is not only in meetings. A lady called Esther saw the anointing on my wife as Chris was simply chatting at a hospital bedside to one of the patients. It's likely that halos were first added to pictures of saints not just to emphasize their holiness but because the anointing had been seen upon them. And photographs have demonstrated how the electro-magnetic field around a person's hands and body alters significantly during a period of ministry.

Chris once asked the Lord to pervade her entire body. Her fervent desire was that he should possess every component, and she found herself naming each one. Some years later we were ministering to a handicapped girl when Esther saw something she felt was so awesome that she couldn't bring herself to share it for several days. Then she told us how, as my wife had been ministering to the girl, Chris's face had undergone a remarkable transformation and become the face of Jesus.

How the anointing helps

The anointing is bound to make a difference to a Christian's life and ministry, and other people will be watching to see that difference (Acts 10:32–39).

IT BRINGS ASSURANCE

When Queen Elizabeth II was anointed with oil at her coronation it was not only for the particular responsibilities she faced but in recognition that she was Queen.

When Christ (which means anointed one) was anointed with the Holy Spirit after his baptism it was not only for the ministry he would exercise but in recognition that he was God's Son—'A voice came from heaven: "You are my Son, whom I love; with you I am well pleased"' (Lk 3:21–23). John the Baptist also saw the anointing on Jesus in the form of a dove, and said, 'I have seen and testify that this is the Son of God' (Jn 1:32–34).

Sometimes God anoints a Christian simply because the Father loves to bless his sons and daughters (Rom 8:15–16). Occasionally Chris and I receive fresh anointings after ministering, either just to assure us of his love or to refill us with his power. Sometimes the anointing is one confirmation that we're doing the right thing. When we had applied to buy a house in Tonbridge, Chris and I knew that because of our faith ministry it wouldn't be easy to obtain a mortgage. But many were praying, and we ourselves joined hands and agreed together for the mortgage at the exact time that it was being negotiated (Mt 18:19). As we did we both felt the Lord's anointing drop upon us. The mortgage was soon granted, with no strings attached, and our building society manager commented that this was 'quite remarkable', as they had never had a case like it.

It brings awareness

God's anointing on our lives is also bound to make a difference to the way we see things. Music directed by him can be another means of releasing healing energy—'While the harpist was playing, the hand of the Lord came upon Elisha' (2 Kings 3:15). It was under the anointing in this context of worship that the prophet was inspired to share some specific and significant revelations.

When the anointing is upon us we may be able to see people and circumstances in a different light. During the Canadian revival anointed believers were able to ascertain just by looking at people 'those who were in victory and those who were not'.

IT BRINGS ACTIVITY

The Lord's anointing enables us to be freer and bolder in our worship and witness. When we have the opportunity to minister God's word we see more spiritual fruit, for there's power in that word when it's proclaimed under the anointing. 'Were not our hearts burning within us,' asked two disciples, 'while he talked with us on the road and opened the Scriptures to us?' (Lk 24:32).

A more recent Christian, Lewi Pethrus, spoke with such power and authority that everyone present automatically rose and worshipped the Lord when he had finished preaching. The anointing was frequently evident in the way he expounded the Scriptures and dealt with evil.

To be anointed doesn't mean to be so frantically involved in activity that we manifest God's power without his love and guidance. He doesn't want us to burn out for him but to burn on for him (Rom 12:11).

Where the anointing leads

IT LEADS TO SERVICE

'God anointed Jesus of Nazareth with the Holy Spirit and power, and . . . he went around doing good and healing all who were under the power of the devil, because God was with him' (Acts 10:38). While the anointing is not only for service, it's especially to equip us for this.

Jesus wasn't anointed after his baptism to make him a child of God, nor to make him holy or sinless—he already was all of these. It was especially to give him power to do God's work. In the same way the anointing doesn't automatically make right our relationship with God or make us holy, but it gives us power to do the works that Jesus did (Jn 14:12).

So what Christ was anointed to do, we are empowered to do—'The Spirit of the Lord is on me, because he has anointed me to preach good news to the poor. He has sent me to proclaim freedom for the prisoners and recovery of sight for the blind, to release the oppressed, to proclaim the year of the Lord's favour' (Lk 4:18–19).

We may be anointed to do particular tasks. One lady was called to be 'an opener of doors and an unblocker of ears'. Sometimes Christians are anointed to prepare them for specific ministry. One day Chris felt her face harden. 'What does it mean?' she asked me.

'Well, the only thing I can think of is when Jesus set his face like a flint to go to Jerusalem,' I replied thoughtfully (Lk 9:51). It transpired that Chris was to see through determinedly a four-day fast while we were delivering a girl from evil spirits.

When someone is too shy to minister healing we can encourage him to pray for the anointing as this can give him confidence. He will still need to step out in faith, but if he gets spiritual stage-fright and requires a prompter the Holy Spirit will be waiting in the wings to reassure him. Jesus' promise to the persecuted is equally applicable to those who minister healing—'Do not worry about what to say or how to say it. At that time you will be given what to say, for it will not be you speaking, but the Spirit of your Father speaking through you' (Mt 10:19–20).

Three types of leader anointed with oil for their tasks were the prophet, priest and king. Jesus is our prophet, priest and king, but we have seen how his anointing was with the Holy Spirit and power (Acts 10:38). It's for this reason that anointing with oil is a symbol of the Holy Spirit's influence and linked with gifts of healing from the same Spirit (1 Cor 12:9). Olive oil was already used in medical treatment and first-aid (Lk 10:34), but nowadays it's especially utilized in the healing ministry to believers.

James wrote, 'Is any one of you sick? He should call the

elders of the church to pray over him and anoint him with oil in the name of the Lord' (Jas 5:14). This is especially appropriate for housebound believers, but we also read that when the twelve apostles first went out 'they anointed many sick people with oil and healed them' (Mk 6:13). Today there are many instances of people being healed through this means. A famous entertainer's son fell over a cliff and was unconscious with a pierced lung, but a pastor anointed the boy with oil in Jesus' name and he recovered.

Chris and I only tend to use oil with specific individuals when the Lords shows us to. We then ask him to bless it for his service, and make the sign of the cross on the forehead of the sick person concerned (Ps 23:5). This ministry is different from extreme unction where the purpose is to prepare someone for death. Anointing with oil can help restore someone to life. It's possible to anoint with oil while knowing nothing of the anointing of the Spirit, but if we also experience the latter we will see more doors unlocked that lead to wholeness.

IT LEADS TO SUFFERING

John the Baptist promised that Christ would 'baptise you with the Holy Spirit and with fire' (Mt 3:11). From the moment we're baptized in the Spirit the powers of darkness will seek us out. If we walk in the light we will be all right (1 Jn 1:7), but anointed Christians often find themselves in the forefront of the battle and take the full force of the Enemy's attacks. After his anointing 'Jesus was led by the Spirit into the desert to be tempted by the devil' (Mt 4:1). And after he had proclaimed the message of healing in his home town the people tried to throw him down the cliff (Lk 4:29).

It's especially when we leave words for actions that opposition follows. William Wilberforce encountered far more opposition once he not only talked about abolishing the slave trade but introduced measures to do so. Believers with anointed ministries who are constantly in the forefront of spiritual warfare are prime targets for the Enemy—that's why they need particular prayer backing.

But in spite of the cost anointed Christians are often victorious Christians. For the anointing is not just a rocket to get us off the ground—it gives us power to maintain a correct course. If we remain under the anointing we not only advance along well-used pathways but we can 'make a track where others have not trod'.

IT LEADS TO SURRENDER

Anointed Christians tend to be out-and-out Christians, white-hot for the Lord (Rev 3:15). Of all electrical appliances it's the ones utilized for heating that use most power. And when we see believers anointed with power we can expect heat—that is, vision and passion—to be prominent in their lives.

Unction cannot be earned, only received—'You have an anointing from the Holy One' (1 Jn 2:20). It's received through prayer and moving in the Spirit. Ignorance, pride, fear or unbelief can prevent us from receiving the Lord's anointing, but if we surrender these to Jesus we can be equipped afresh, with or without the laying-on-of-hands.

It's humbling for people who have been Christians for many years to come back to the source of supply, but that's what we sometimes have to do. A village had once lost all its community spirit, but then a drought arose and everyone had to go back to the village pump. There at that source of supply a community spirit quickly grew again and affected the whole village.

Finally, having received the anointing, we need to rest under it. Another secret of an effective healing ministry is adopting a sailing-ship lifestyle instead of a rowing-boat one. If we struggle with the oars of our own strength we'll soon become discouraged and defeated, but if we abide under the Lord's anointing (1 Jn 2:27) and allow the wind of the Holy Spirit to blow us along we'll advance further and be more encouraged. There will still be work to do on board but we won't be in charge of it.

So this built-in central heating is available to all who mean business with God. And according to how much we avail ourselves of all this power—the dynamite, the authority and the anointing—thus powerful will we be in bringing Jesus' healing to the world (Acts 1:8).

Suggested reading: Luke 4:14–30.

Key 6

CHANGE: THE KEY TO CHRISTIAN PROGRESS

18

Choose Your Rut Carefully

In certain remote areas of Australia there are no proper roads so motorists have to drive in the ruts. Every so often they meet a sign—'Choose your rut carefully—you'll be in it for the next forty miles.'

Sometimes we Christians have chosen our ruts so carefully that we're in danger of remaining in them for the next forty years. But healing may only take place when we move out of our ruts and on with the Lord.

A willingness to change

At the pool of Bethesda Jesus healed only one man because that man turned his eyes away from the pool and onto the Lord (Jn 5:1–8). Jesus asked him first, 'Do you want to get well? That may sound a strange question to ask someone who has been an invalid for thirty-eight years, but some people have decided subconsciously that they will be sick or die, while others prefer to remain ill and be nursed or mollycoddled. When Christians ministered to a blind lady in Ireland she began to see specks of light, but then she became frightened and said, 'Please don't pray for me any more.' Perhaps she couldn't cope with the prospect of being able to see clearly (contrast Mk 8:23–25).

Sick people must be willing to receive ministry, so we offer it but don't force it. Even when people reject the offer it may still have been right to have made it, for it shows them we care, and they may approach us at some other time. Sick folk must usually respond to the ministry as best they can, at least by following our prayers in their minds.

You cannot reason with hedgehogs—they curl up into a ball, but you may be able to help a bird to fly if it really wants to. Similarly, when a person is unwilling to be helped, we can only pray that the Holy Spirit will convict him of his need (Jn 16:8), for we can only help those who desire our ministry. But the more a sick person wants to be healed, the easier it usually is to help him.

However, a person who is unwilling to receive ministry may come to that point later on, perhaps when he is desperate. If he doesn't respond immediately we don't keep on at him. Fruit trees left alone a year often fruit far better the following year, and sometimes we have to wait before we see any fruit in a particular situation.

F. B. Meyer once confessed, 'Lord, I'm not willing, but I'm willing to be made willing.' We all fear change to some extent, but those of us who minister also have to be willing for radical changes in our hearts which means taking one step forward at a time with the Lord.

Letting go of the past

Naaman the leper was furious. 'Go, wash yourself seven times in the Jordan,' he had been told (2 Kings 5:10–11). His reaction was 'Isn't there some other way for me to be healed? Can't I bathe in my own rivers?' But he had consulted the Lord's prophet so his healing had to be on the

Lord's terms. It was only when he let go of his own ideas, obeyed, and came up out of the water the seventh time that his flesh 'became clean like that of a young boy' (2 Kings 5:14).

Before a person is physically or mentally healed he may have to let go of something. God may be waiting for him to be born again, be baptized, or take some other step before the healing is manifested. Sometimes God may wait for those who minister healing to let go of the past in a specific way before he will use them fully. Chris and I had to come to the point where we were ready to sacrifice our ministries if that was the only way to go forward with Jesus.

Watchman Nee believed that part of the normal Christian life was to be 'crucified with Christ' (Gal 2:20). A young man once asked an old saint, 'What does it mean to be crucified?'

'Well,' he replied, 'the crucified person's facing only one direction. If he hears anything behind him he can't turn round to see what's going on. Also he's not going back—when you go out to die on a cross you say goodbye. And he has no further plans of his own—somebody else makes his plans for him, and when they nail him up there all his plans disappear.'

When Bartimaeus heard Jesus approaching he threw off his yellow cloak, the symbol of his old life of blindness—comparable in those days to a white stick or a guide dog. Jesus told him, before he could even see, 'Your faith has healed you.' So Bartimaeus became one of the few Bible characters we know of who, after being healed by Christ, followed him (Mk 10:50–52).

The extent to which people can let go of their past depends on how firm a hold something has upon them. Short grass can be pulled up easily, but dandelions are slightly harder to remove because they have a deeper root. Some weeds seem to lift off the ground easily but underneath the roots have spread, while prickly thistles are so deeply fixed that they are often the most difficult to uproot. In the same way people can easily give over to the Lord some things from their past, but other things have a greater hold upon them, and before they can make progress they may require ministry for these things.

LOOSING THE BONDS

Like many Christians I can sing with rejoicing those words of Charles Wesley, 'My chains fell off, my heart was free!' But every so often the Lord says, 'John, you're getting bound to something again and you need to be set free.' And I cannot move forward very far if I have a heavy chain around me.

Some people are bound to their sicknesses. Jesus said of the woman with the bowed back, 'Satan has kept [her] bound for eighteen long years' (Lk 13:16). Other people are harmfully tied to negative attitudes or circumstances. We can encourage them to picture the chains falling away as we cut them free in Jesus' name (Jn 8:32). But they must be willing to let go of their bondages.

Those who possess occult books or charms need to destroy them (Acts 19:19). A Christian lady called Lilian was given a Christmas present which turned out to be an idol. 'What should I do with it?' she asked.

'Destroy it!' Chris and I replied. Although the person who gave it probably intended no harm, it had been dedicated to another god and therefore Satan could use it to bring Lilian into bondage.

Many folk are harmfully bound to other people, especially loved ones, authority figures, and others who have influenced them. When ministering Chris and I thank God for the helpful ties and cords of love, and we pray that all good influences from these people will remain in the sufferer, but we set him free from those who have power over him in his mind. We may only be able to do this at his end of the chain, but it enables him to be free to relate to them or think of them in a new way and to act and react differently as a result (Gal 5:1). He may even be bound to the dead, perhaps still suffering from an inferiority complex because of a dominating parent who is now deceased. But as we set him free from this parent, or his ancestral line, he can find a new liberty (Lk 4:18).

Fear is something else that binds us. Sometimes we're afraid to be blessed, yet God would appreciate it if we gave him permission to bless us. Sometimes we're afraid to show it if we are blessed. At other times we're frightened of letting people down, or afraid we won't keep to what we've promised. An alcoholic stumbled into one of our meetings, and when he had sobered up he was overcome with conviction of sin. Chris and I led him to accept Jesus as his Saviour, but then he became worried that he wouldn't be able to keep up being a Christian because of his drinking problem. We assured him that Jesus would give him the power—he just had to be willing.

Many of us stay in our secret prisons, not daring to open up and share because we're so afraid as Christians that our own failings will be exposed in the process. A Christian whom I'll call woman A woke up in the night and saw a picture of a key. God said he would show her the key to woman B's problems—it was woman C. Woman A would never have guessed that woman C was responsible, yet woman B had known and had been afraid to share it. Until such people as woman B are released from the bondage of fear they will make little progress in receiving or sharing healing, for fear causes disease and hinders convalescence.

It's particularly difficult sometimes to step out in faith where we're well known—at home, at work, or even in our own churches, because we fear the people we're constantly involved with and what they will think. The best answer may be to receive afresh through the laying-on-of-hands the perfect love of Jesus which casts out fear (1 Jn 4:18). Whether it's a mental attitude or an evil spirit of fear, we can be released from it if we're willing to let it go and look to him.

Our old selfish natures can also bring us into bondage, and some Christians find it helpful to bind their imaginations before praying. Paul wrote, 'We take captive every thought to make it obedient to Christ' (2 Cor 10:5). Part of the healing process is the renewing of the mind (Rom 12:2).

Sometimes Christians try casting out what they should be crucifying in themselves (Rom 6:11). Samuel Chadwick was honest enough to burn fifteen 'perfect' sermons because 'there was too much of the flesh in them'. He didn't realize just how dry they were until he set light to them.

Another of Naaman's problems was his pride. He was enraged because he wasn't given instant healing by the prophet Elisha in person (2 Kings 5:11). Many people are finding they need to let go of their pride and self-consciousness before they are healed or can make progress. A minister who had been unsympathetic to signs and wonders attended a healing meeting and afterwards admitted he had to reconsider his views. This helped him to overcome his stubbornness and pride. But false modesty can also become a chain around us, for constantly emphasizing our inadequacy and unworthiness can be an inverted form of pride.

Our traditions, even the good ones, can also bind us if we rigidly adhere to them without being open to the Holy Spirit, and our worship can become so stereotyped that the Lord is thoroughly bored with it. If we overemphasize particular doctrines, such as discipleship, submission, or prosperity, we can become entangled in as much bondage as those involved in legalistic systems like Jehovah's Witnesses, the Moonies, or Scientology. Involvement with Freemasonry always tends to stunt real spiritual growth, and pseudo-Christian sects and cults attract religious evil spirits whose task is to bring people into bondage (Col 2:18–23). But just as strong are the chains forged by some Christian churches that have a remarkable ability to absorb new movements of the Holy Spirit and neutralize them.

The other main area of bondage lies in habits and compulsive addictions. Whenever anyone entered a particular lady's home she would prevent them from sitting down until she had flicked every speck of dust off all the cushions. Then she would apologize profusely, 'Sorry, sorry. My late husband was allergic to dust and I can't get out of the habit.'

Jesus can break the chains of habit and addiction: to drugs, sexual perversion, violence, gambling, drinking and smoking. Joe is a Yorkshireman who went forward at a meeting to be baptized in the Holy Spirit. During the service he showed no evidence of new release, but when he left the building and lit a cigarette it tasted bitter and he couldn't smoke it. God had delivered him from bondage to nicotine, and he kept free of the addiction.

One of the results of charismatic renewal has been a release from inhibitions. In our own meetings people can feel free: to speak, sing, clap hands, dance, raise their hands in worship, or to do none of these things. When we're not free we may need to come to the point where firstly we can accept ourselves as we are, and secondly we can accept what Jesus wants to make us.

Meanwhile, when we minister freedom we shouldn't forget to let loose the Holy Spirit's power (Mt 18:18) and if necessary to reinforce a deliverance several times until the person concerned discovers that his chains have vanished completely.

LEAVING THE BURDENS

A butterfly once kept trying to get out of my vicarage

study through a closed window. There was an open window nearby but the butterfly persisted in assaulting the closed one.

Many people are striving to get rid of their problems when what they need to do is leave them with Jesus. Another rendering of Matthew 11:28 is 'Come to me all in labour, and I will relieve you.' Augustine said, 'Thou hast made us for thyself, and our hearts are restless until they find their rest in thee.'

Healing doesn't usually come through striving, and it doesn't only come through intense ministry. One beautiful summer's evening Chris and I were walking under the trees on Tunbridge Wells common. 'Doesn't it minister to you!' she exclaimed. Her choice of word seemed entirely appropriate. A therapist once remarked, 'What I do is provide the right environment and allow the body to heal.'

Those who are constantly planning for the future find it difficult not to 'worry about tomorrow' (Mt 6:34) and only live one day at a time. Some of us are like elastic bands stretched to their limit at both ends. Because we fear losing control of a situation we become too tense to receive anything, let alone healing. Naaman had to give in, and it's never easy to do that, but if we're willing the Lord can relax us inside.

A man who kept a tight rein on himself received through ministry a spirit of casualness and carefree abandon. As he believed he had received this (Mk 11:24), and endeavoured to take life more easily, he became a different person.

A woman was struggling with a sack of potatoes when a lorry driver offered her a lift. On arriving at the woman's house he opened the back door of the lorry to let her out. There she stood, still shouldering her sack of potatoes.

When we're unable to cope with a situation we not only need to give our burdens over to the Lord but to leave them there. Satan will try to pile weights upon us but as we lay aside every weight, as well as our sin, and keep our eyes fixed on Jesus (Heb 12:1–2) we'll find healing. When Peter wrote, 'Cast all your anxiety upon him' (1 Pet 5:7), he was describing a deliberate action, and used the same word for 'cast' as the one used when the disciples threw their cloaks over the donkey Jesus rode on the first Palm Sunday (Mk 11:7).

Some Christians find it helpful to write down their problems, place their hands on what they have written as they offer it to the Lord, then either burn the paper or write down when the burdens are lifted.

LIFTING THE BARRIERS

At some level-crossings all the motorist has to do is sit in his car and wait until the barriers are lifted. At others he must get out of his vehicle and open the gates himself. When we're conscious of barriers in our lives we can sometimes only wait trustfully until they are lifted, but frequently we can play a part in removing them.

Before a barrier can be removed it must be recognized, and that may mean looking behind why people act as they do. When a man died, apparently suddenly, his son Roger grew bitter as a result. But then Roger talked to the doctor to find out more, and learned that his father had really been ill for twenty years. Roger then saw things in a different light, realizing that God had added twenty years to his father's life (compare 2 Kings 20:6).

Sometimes people put up barriers by thoughtlessness, like the butler who forgot all about Joseph in prison (Gen 40:23) and therefore delayed the healing of Joseph's circumstances. At other times people have subconscious barriers. While those ministering only need to deal with what surfaces or what they are led to, if someone is aware he has a barrier but doesn't know what it is, this may need to be shared and prayed about.

Two other factors are relevant here. One is to avoid

negative thoughts even in jest, for our subconscious minds don't know when we're kidding. The other is that when someone gets worse before being healed, God may be bringing the bad things to the surface and lifting them out of the sufferer.

Once a barrier has been recognized it needs to be repented of.

Why is it that Elisha could raise a dead boy but Gehazi his servant couldn't? (2 Kings 4:31–35). One reason was because Gehazi was deceitful (2 Kings 5:20–22)—his heart wasn't right before God and he needed to repent. We Christians also need to repent—of the unbelief in our churches which has made us an unbelieving nation, and of whatever is holding back our spiritual progress (Rev 3:19).

Part of the healing ministry is encouraging others to repent (Mk 6:12–13). Once again, it's especially when we minister that we see things happen. Counsellors have noticed that there's often more repentance expressed in the prayer than in the talking beforehand.

The keys to healing can actually have the effect of locking doors if turned the wrong way—that is, if the people receiving the benefits of them resist them. It sometimes takes time for people to go completely in the direction that the Lord is leading. It took God 430 years to get the Israelites out of slavery in Egypt (Ex 12:40–41). It then took him another forty years to get Egyptian customs out of the children of Israel (Ps 95:10). When sinners do repent, however, there's joy not only for them but in heaven (Lk 15:7, 10). Once when this happened in a house group the Lord said, 'I've a few angels around me right now and we're all rejoicing.'

If we maintain barriers in our churches the Lord won't push through them. He'll move aside like a gentleman and go where people are open to him. But he longs to put things right because he loves us. When Paul wrote about equipping the saints for ministry (Eph 4:12 RSV) he used a word which means setting bones back into their proper place. Jesus wants to heal his body the church by putting things back into their correct position, and that will only happen as we let him do what he wants to in our lives.

A man was once healed of pain in his back, stomach and joints, but wondered why he still couldn't move his neck. At another meeting he heard the Lord calling him to full surrender (Rom 12:1), and the healing was completed.

I can come to Jesus just as I am, but I do need to let go of the past if I want to go on with him (Col 2:6)—unless, of course, I've chosen my rut rather too carefully.

Suggested readings: 2 Kings 5:1–14; Luke 13:10–17.

19

The 'Whether' Forecast

'The outlook for tomorrow is showers with bright periods . . . and that's the end of the weather forecast.'

The outlook for us and those we minister healing to also depends to some extent on a 'whether' forecast—whether we'll trust the Lord not only to release us from our past but to take charge of our future, and whether we'll go forward step by step in obedience to him.

Letting God take the future

Because the future is so uncertain, and because we like to control our own destiny, we hesitate to let God take responsibility for what's to come. Yet part of the healing ministry is helping people to give their unknown future into his healing hands (Ps 31:5).

At one of our conferences I was asked, 'What should I do if I'm to be operated on by a surgeon of another religion?'

I replied, 'Go ahead and trust the Lord to take care of you.' It's never easy to go under an anaesthetic, especially for a major operation, but we have to put our trust in many people whose backgrounds we know little of. If you believe you're doing the right thing by having an operation, and if you ensure that Christians are backing you up in prayer, you can not only know that God will take care of you but you're likely to experience his very real peace (Phil 4:6–7).

Another area where we need to let God take the future is that of travel. Although the number of road accidents in our country is appallingly high, many must have been averted because Christians bothered to pray. Chris and I were once travelling up the M11 motorway to take a teaching day in Norfolk when we saw seven or eight damaged vehicles strewn along the side of the road. Had we reached there a few minutes earlier we would almost certainly have been involved in the pile-up that had taken place, and we were very conscious of the prayers of those who were remembering us.

When we do encounter setbacks the important thing is not to get hung up on failure or withdraw from our circumstances but to make a fresh start. When Chris and I first took up horse riding we noticed that riders who came off their horses and were badly shaken up usually mounted them again straight away, thus minimizing the fears and anxieties that might have arisen as a result of the shock.

When we get thrown off balance in our Christian lives or find ourselves slipping backwards the devil will whisper that it's no use going on. But if we let the Lord pick us up again and start us off afresh, and if we get involved in ministry to others we'll soon find we're making spiritual progress once more. 'Forgetting what is behind and straining towards what is ahead, I press on towards the goal' (Phil 3:13–14).

LEARNING TO BE LED

When Saul of Tarsus came off his horse, on the road to

Damascus, he was temporarily blinded and had the humiliating experience of having to be 'led by the hand' (Acts 9:8).

As we let Jesus take us by the hand he will lead us wherever he wants us to go. Chris and I once prayed, 'Lord, we'll do anything for you, we'll go anywhere with you.' This was a dangerous prayer to pray because God took us at our word, and through many painful experiences he moulded us and trained us for the ministry into which he eventually led us.

A similar sort of prayer is necessary for those who would make progress in the healing ministry, for the supreme test of our ministering healing is the place the Lord occupies in it. Is he really put in charge? Does he decide things, or is he only called upon to help carry out the plans of others?

We cannot walk in the flesh and the Spirit at the same time (Gal 5:16), and only what's done in the Spirit will last (1 Cor 3:10–15). This means following in the steps of Jesus. It's extremely difficult to place our feet into the exact footprints of someone who has gone ahead, but if that same person is also walking beside us to hold our hands it's made much easier.

When the brilliant light suddenly flashed around Saul on the Damascus road 'he fell to the ground' (Acts 9:4), and it was there in the lowest place that he began to learn to be led.

Sometimes God has to bring people to the lowest place, but it's from there that he can really do something with them. Jonah had a genuine change of heart once he was in the belly of the whale (Jon 2:1–2), and Joseph could only look in one direction from the bottom of the pit—upwards (Gen 37:23–24).

However, Jesus said to Saul, 'Get up' (Acts 9:6), and he 'got up from the ground' (Acts 9:8). In the field of healing we cannot make 'humility' an excuse for staying where we are. We have to stand and be ready to follow the Lord.

When Saul got up he opened his eyes but could see nothing (Acts 9:8). He had to wait for three days before he could see again (Acts 9:9). As for having light on what to do, he had been given just the first step by Jesus—'Go into the city, and you will be told what you must do' (Acts 9:6).

The Lord doesn't always give us light on all we're to do for him, and often he shows us just one step at a time. If we keep on asking him the next step should become clear (Mt 7:7). However, the Lord tends to work in seasons, and Chris and I have had periods, sometimes each lasting several months, when our guidance has been clearcut, while during others we've walked in the dark.

Some Christians when challenged about someone in need always answer, 'I'll pray about it.' The Lord knows whether they really do. Making progress in healing ministry means seeking God's light on situations and sharing it when opportunity arises with those who may desperately require it (Prov 13:17).

After Saul's conversion his ministry was limited at first to the city of Damascus (Acts 9:19–22). Similarly, we have seen how God has particular people he desires us to minister to and particular areas he will lead us into. We will be most effective when we keep to those situations he has prepared for us.

Once someone has been ill, even if he is completely healed, he may have a weak spot in the area of his body or mind where he was affected and may need to watch the source of his problem so it doesn't arise again. In the same way God knows our limitations and wants us to bear these in mind. If someone attends one or two training days, for instance, or reads a book like this, it doesn't mean he knows all there is to know about healing and can minister it anyhow—he needs to be led.

We have also seen how the Lord leads us in varying

ways on different occasions in the areas he calls us to. The house groups I've been involved with have often been led to minister in their meetings in different ways. Sometimes the leaders alone might lay hands on people present. Sometimes the group might join hands in a circle and allow the Lord's healing power to flow through to one another. Other times they might split into smaller groups. Then again someone present might be given a prophecy indicating the Lord's way for ministering at that particular meeting.

On the other hand, Saul's ministry didn't remain confined to Damascus. In the Lord's way and time it extended to the farthest limits of the known world. Let's pursue the vision God gives us as it widens, while keeping in step with him and so being prepared for any eventuality wherever we may be.

Dave and Jackie are one of many couples I've been training, and Jackie has been especially used in counselling. But one day when they were in a supermarket and a girl fainted, Jackie automatically found herself putting her training into action by kneeling on the floor, laying hands on the girl and praying for her (see Eph 5:16).

LEARNING TO BE FED

Another immediate result of Saul's first encounter with Jesus was that 'for three days he . . . did not eat or drink anything' (Acts 9:9). He knew what it was to go without. Chris and I tell in *It Hurts to Heal* of some occasions when we've had to go without. Once all we had in our house was beetroot, and I don't like beetroot. It's doubtful if we can appreciate the needs of some people unless we ourselves have also gone without. This doesn't mean we allow Satan to rob us of those good things Jesus desires for us (Jn 10:1, 10), for part of healing is when the Lord restores what has been lost through wasted years (Joel 2:25–26).

Eventually Saul was healed, filled with the Spirit and

baptized (Acts 9:17–18), 'and after taking some food, he regained his strength' (Acts 9:19). He was learning to be fed by those he had previously opposed and this enabled him to grow spiritually at a rapid rate.

In the same way we are to become like little children (Mt 18:3), but we shouldn't stay like that. As we feed upon the Lord we can progress from milk to solid food, and 'solid food is for the mature, who by constant use have trained themselves to distinguish good from evil' (Heb 5:14). Doctors believe that crash diets are unhelpful —it's better to diet slowly over a period. We cannot digest all our spiritual food in one helping, nor force it down the throats of those who cannot take it, but the food is available to those who desire it.

At a teaching day a lady asked, 'Won't it be selfish, when I know of others who are sick, if I have ministry for my own healing?'

I replied, 'No, it's your right—not because of anything you've done but because it's part of the inheritance Jesus has won for you on the cross' (Is 53:5). Receiving ministry ourselves can be a means by which we are fed by the Lord and built up in him.

We are all at different stages of spiritual growth. I may be ahead of some of you in certain areas of the healing ministry but you can probably teach me much in other areas.

'Saul spent several days with the disciples in Damascus' (Acts 9:19) and so began to gain experience of Christian fellowship. Only when we experience something can we really speak with authority about it, and teachers cannot assume that if something has been taught once it's necessarily been thoroughly digested.

In the healing ministry we especially need to grow in experience of people, and we can never really know a person by how he thinks, only by how he feels. The different terms Jesus uses for his disciples indicate how their relationship with him was progressing. First he calls them servants (Jn 13:13–16), later friends (Jn 15:14–15), and finally brothers (Jn 20:17–18).

LEARNING TO BE BLED

Regularity is a sign of fitness, while irregular bodily functions indicate a person is unhealthy. Another aspect of letting God take the future is discipline. The word 'discipline' comes from the same root as 'discipleship'. It includes regular attention to God's will for us and how we can achieve it (Eph 5:17). It also means counting the cost. We shouldn't attempt to take on what we don't mean to follow through (Lk 14:28–33). How far are we ready to cope with the results of healing ministry, or to be moulded by the Lord through times of trial? If we're praying for revival we also need to pray we'll be ready to cope with the riots that inevitably follow it (Acts 8:1).

The church is at its weakest when it is 'at ease in Zion' (Amos 6:1 AV)—affluent, complacent and self-sufficient. It is at its strongest when under persecution, like the enslaved Israelites were—'The more they were oppressed, the more they multiplied and spread; so the Egyptians came to dread the Israelites' (Ex 1:12).

Saul was left in no doubt that his ministry wouldn't be easy—'I will show him how much he must suffer for my name' (Acts 9:16). It looks as if Jesus disclosed to him a 'video' of the stonings, lashings, imprisonments, shipwrecks and other perils to come (2 Cor 11:24–29).

In spite of this, many years later Paul's greatest ambition was still 'I want to know Christ and the power of his resurrection and the fellowship of sharing in his sufferings, becoming like him in his death' (Phil 3:10). So to be like Jesus in ministering healing means not just in character and service but in becoming 'acquainted with grief' as he was (Is 53:3 RSV). It means having our hearts broken by the same things that broke his heart. A lady found herself crying each time she interceded for the sick. Jesus was allowing her to experience something of the fellowship of his sufferings, not just what he suffered on the cross (Col 1:24) but the suffering he experiences today as his heart bleeds for sick and needy people.

Ministering healing involves the sacrifice of praise (Heb 13:15) and the sacrifice of prayer (Heb 5:7). It may mean getting up in the middle of the night to minister to the dying, but such sacrifice can mean the difference between someone going to be with the Lord or not (Jn 3:18). A dying person may hear you long after he has ceased to be able to communicate with you, therefore you could be God's agent in bringing him the greatest healing of all.

Jean is another Christian lady who has attended our training days, and she has experienced the physical pain that sometimes follows when we sacrifice ourselves in the service of Jesus. Once she saw fiery darts coming at her from all sides (Eph 6:16) and suffered intense pain, but the Lord said to her, 'Use my name!' and when she did the attack ceased. Such experiences haven't discouraged Jean, rather they've encouraged her to serve the Lord even more. On another occasion, while ministering to a lady aged eighty-six, the Lord said, 'Get to the source.' The woman had back trouble and one leg proved to be shorter than the other. As Jean held her foot and prayed, the smaller leg shot out to the same length as the other. Jean couldn't stop laughing at the suddenness of what the Lord had done.

It's often easy to have all the right words when things are going well, but, when it comes to the crunch, not to be wholehearted. But if our commitment is total, we'll become not just whole but holy. Something the Lord has been saying to Christians in the eighties is, 'Be holy, because I am holy' (1 Pet 1:16).

This book has only touched briefly on some aspects of healing ministry. Bodies like the Churches' Council for

Health and Healing are investigating many more. But, while the future of healing in the church seems guaranteed, what sort of future that will be depends largely on the 'whether' forecast—whether ordinary people like you and me are wholehearted in commitment to Jesus.

Suggested reading: Acts 9:1–22.

20

Launch out into the Deep

If we let go of the past and let God take the future, we will be ready to launch out in the present in healing ministry.

Launching out in the present

One day when Simon Peter and his fishing crew had worked hard all night with no success (Lk 5:5), Jesus said to Peter, 'Launch out into the deep, and let down your nets' (Lk 5:4 AV). They obeyed him and 'caught such a large number of fish that their nets began to break' (Lk 5:6).

WHAT DOES IT MEAN TO LAUNCH?

In the Bible the deep sometimes symbolizes the place of hazards. Somebody once remarked to me, 'The book of Revelation states that in God's new heaven and earth there'll be no more sea (Rev 21:1). Isn't that a shame, for the sea's such a beautiful part of his creation?'

But I replied, 'Don't worry, it simply means there'll be no more trouble, and no more need for healing. Verse 4 of the same chapter says, "He will wipe away every tear from their eyes. There will be no more death or mourning or crying or pain."'

Launching out into the deep may therefore mean venturing into troubled waters. It doesn't mean deliberately searching for trouble, but it does mean going with Jesus into situations where healing is required and which could prove costly and difficult. In these situations we need to be aware of any dangers, just as the look-out on a ship scans the horizon for rocks, icebergs, large sea creatures or other vessels.

The deep also symbolizes the place of harvest, for it's only in deep waters that big fish are caught. Launching out into the deep therefore means going into situations where people are ready to be brought to the Lord and through our ministry find their needs met in him (Acts 14:9–10).

So it's dangerous in the deep waters but it's exciting and fulfilling. And if we launch out the Lord will ensure that our heads are kept above water.

Launching out entails making the most of opportunities for healing. We have already seen how Jesus was expert at launching into healing. Whether he was faced with a comparatively simple need or one requiring a miracle, immediately it was time to minister he would step out in faith by opening his mouth to speak or reaching out his hand to touch. We have also seen how his power and gifts can enable us to do the same. So when one young man I read about had the opportunity to minister he didn't hesitate but launched out declaring, 'If Jesus can do it, so can I!' (Phil 4:13).

But launching isn't a once-for-all experience—we may need to launch out again and again. If we do, though, we will have God's peace about it and find it gives us confidence to launch still further. A Christian lady launched out by making occasional remarks to a neighbour about the Lord, apparently with no response. But after ten years that neighbour became ill, and the first person she thought of going to for help was the Christian lady.

Something else launching out may mean is encouraging people who have been healed through our ministry to witness to what God has done (Mk 5:19). Many of them won't need to be reminded, but some may hold back because, for instance, Jesus sometimes told people not to mention that he had healed them (Mk 1:44). We have to understand that Jesus probably said this because the time had not yet come for him to openly proclaim that he was the Messiah (Jn 2:4; contrast Mk 14:61–62). He could easily have been strung up on the cross long before God's appointed time if he hadn't warned people about what they might say, especially in those areas (most places) where it could spell danger for him.

Once he had given his great commission (Mk 16:15), however, there were no such restrictions. Words like 'hesitation' and 'reservation' weren't in the vocabulary of the early Christians, while 'boldness' and 'fearlessness' were (Acts 9:27–28). We can be like them as we launch out in the power of the Spirit (Acts 4:31).

Sometimes launching out means helping other believers to go deeper with Jesus and claim the inheritance he has won for them (Eph 1:18). Some brothers and sisters need help to receive the fullness of the Holy Spirit and appropriate it (Acts 8:15–17). Part of the ministry may also include helping Christians to turn their eyes off church structures and administration alone and onto the deeper waters and more important ministries like evangelism and healing. But, while some people quickly respond to this challenge, we need to be patient with others who are slower to accept it.

I can especially understand such people as in my family I'm usually the last to get hold of anything: whether it's seeing the point of a joke, recognizing that something is different about a room, or even catching a cold.

Many years ago when I returned to England on a troopship after doing national service in Singapore, I spotted Southampton as a speck in the distance. Then very gradually the coastline loomed larger, till after a while I could pick out the buildings, the traffic and the pedestrians, and eventually we disembarked and I entered into what I had seen.

Every so often God has shown me something new. At first it's appeared like a speck in the distance, and I've been slow to appreciate its relevance. But then it's gradually made more sense to me, till eventually I've entered into it and made it part of my experience. Jesus is still opening my eyes to new dimensions of healing and wholeness (Lk 24:32; Jn 9:25).

WHY DO WE NEED TO LAUNCH?

There's an urgent need for more of us to launch out into the healing ministry, for more and more people in need are turning to unhelpful sources for healing. A cartoon once portrayed a scene in mid-ocean. Several bedraggled survivors from a shipwreck were clinging to a raft as it surmounted the huge waves. One of the survivors was looking hopeful and pointing. The caption underneath read: 'We're saved! Here comes the Titanic!'

Thousands of people are looking to sinking ships like spiritualism or scientology, many not realizing that Jesus is healing through his church. But 'he is able to save [heal] completely those who come to God through him, because he always lives to intercede for them' (Heb 7:25).

Another cartoon, however, pictured a lone oarsman rowing across the sea and gaily singing while all around him people were drowning. The caption read: 'Hallelujah! I'm bound for Heaven!' Could it be that sometimes we're content to be saved ourselves but oblivious to people very near at hand who are drowning in the effects of sin or sickness?

Some of us who feel more secure on dry land than out in

the deep may also feel more secure by staying where we are rather than launching out with the Lord. Jesus once told a story about a great banquet, and how everyone who was first invited made excuses for not attending. One used his possessions as an excuse, another his work, another his family (Lk 14:18–20). So the organizer of the feast instructed his servants, 'Go out quickly into the streets and alleys of the town and bring in the poor, the crippled, the blind and the lame' (Lk 14:21)—those who needed healing. When this had been done he told his servants, 'Go out to the roads and country lanes and make them come in' (Lk 14:23). There's a sense of urgency about the way so many needy people were not only invited but brought in by the servants to make up the number at the banquet.

Nowadays when the Lord sends his Christian servants to bring sick and needy people to his feast of life and wholeness, it's not only those invited who make excuses, it's sometimes we who are sent. And it's still possessions, work and family that we mention most in this respect. All these may be good in themselves but the Lord wants us to put him first (Mt 6:33), and to launch out when he tells us to.

Sometimes we also put forward more subtle excuses. Perhaps we hold back because we think we're not as good as others at doing a particular task. Moses when challenged to bring Israel out of Egypt said, 'What if they do not believe me?' (Ex 4:1), 'I have never been eloquent' (Ex 4:10), and, 'Please send someone else to do it' (Ex 4:13). He was probably hoping his more eloquent brother Aaron would be chosen. But the Lord never calls us to any task without making available everything we need, and he will equip us if we launch out and take it on (Phil 4:19).

If we rescued a drowning man from the sea we wouldn't leave him to flounder on the shore, we would see he received further assistance. Our motive in launching out into ministry is not just to introduce people to Jesus but to ensure they obtain continuing help for all their needs (Lk 10:35; Philem 17–18).

So we return to wholeness. The deeper we go with Jesus the more we will find ourselves announcing the whole gospel (Rom 15:18–19), ministering to the whole person (1 Thess 5:23), hoping for this in the whole church (Eph 3:14–19), and through it helping to extend God's kingdom through the whole world (Mk 16:15). It's because Paul and his companions launched out so much with Jesus that people exclaimed, 'These men who have turned the world upside down have come here also' (Acts 17:6 Amplified Version).

So what's our ultimate aim in launching out? It's not just the alleviation of physical, mental or emotional needs, speaking to people about Jesus, seeing them converted, ensuring they are filled with the Holy Spirit, nor their becoming faithful members of God's church, nor seeing them witnessing and ministering effectively. Ultimately it is nothing short of their total maturity in Christ (Eph 4:13).

How then do we launch?

The best way to launch into the healing ministry is by making a fresh, deliberate commitment to Jesus that in his power we will go wherever he desires and however deep he calls us to to please him. Then, as we take it for granted we're swimming in deep waters, we'll soon find we are.

Firstly, we should let Jesus give the word. Peter launched at the word of Jesus (Lk 5:4–5). The experienced fisherman didn't question the rabbi's instructions to lower the nets on the 'wrong' side of the ship at the 'wrong' time of day.

Secondly, we should leap into freedom. Peter was taking a leap of faith, just as on another occasion he stepped onto the sea and discovered he could walk on the water all the time he kept his eyes on Jesus (Mt 14:28–29). A leap of faith is a leap into freedom, for the deeper we launch with the Lord the freer we become in ourselves and the more boldness we have to go further.

Most of us, however, begin launching in the shallows. Before Jesus said, 'Launch out into the deep' (Lk 5:4), he had told Peter, 'Put out a little from the shore' (Lk 5:3).

Another man once launched out into the deep by starting in the shallows. His name was Ezekiel. When he stepped into the river that flowed from God's Temple he entered 'water that was ankle-deep' (Ezek 47:3). We don't have to wait until we're deep into the healing ministry before we take our first steps at walking in the Spirit (Gal 5:25).

But, as the Lord is fond of saying to Chris and me, each step is a preparation for the next, and one thing leads to another. Soon the river that Ezekiel was walking in became 'water that was knee-deep' (Ezek 47:4). As we launch deeper into the healing ministry we often learn more about praying in the Spirit (Eph 6:18).

After that Ezekiel was wading in 'water that was up to the waist' (Ezek 47:4). A further stage for us may be resting in the Spirit (Ps 37:7)—learning more to wait on the Lord and relax in him.

Finally 'the water was deep enough to swim in' (Ezek 47:5). When someone is swimming in deep water often only his head can be seen. As we launch stage by stage with Jesus we want to get to the point where, when we minister, people will see Christ our head as pre-eminent (Col 1:18).

Some of us launch out but draw back when we realize what's involved. We start with good intentions but, when the going gets rough, withdraw to a 'safer' situation.

We saw in chapter 4 how we have no need to drop back if our faith isn't big enough for a particular situation where healing is required. We can pray instead within our faith, one step at a time. In certain circumstances we can also pray beyond our faith. If other Christians present can believe for more than we can that doesn't necessarily mean we have to drop out of the race (Gal 5:7). We can pray for those believers and they can minister to the people in need.

As we persevere in prayer (Lk 11:5–8) we will often find our faith increasing (Lk 17:5). As we advance believing that we're equipped we'll find that we are. The more we use the gifts of the Spirit the more they will increase in us. The more we apply the keys to healing the more doors will Jesus open through us.

When it comes to a whole church launching out, it's said that the growth and effectiveness of any fellowship tends to be in direct proportion to its ability to mobilize its members in the task of continuous outreach. So an every-member ministry that is also outward-looking tends to be most effective. And two other things seem necessary in connection with the way churches launch out—reconciliation (Mt 5:23–24) and relevance (1 Cor 9:19–23).

Because Peter's crew had caught so many fish 'they signalled their partners in the other boat to come and help them' (Lk 5:7). This is the attitude that aids healing ministry among the churches—not competition or confrontation but co-operation. At Breath Fellowship meetings people are usually unaware of the denominations to which people sitting next to them owe allegiance. We forget our labels as we seek to go forward together, 'all one in Christ Jesus' (Gal 3:28).

Our different denominations are like separate ponds with ducks on each that can easily be identified. But when the floods of the Holy Spirit come in, the water from each pond runs into the others till all the ducks get mixed up and are swimming around together.

Many Christians hope that this will happen more. Not that we gloss over our differences, but that we make them subservient to our main task.

The other need is that we make our ministry relevant to the person in the street. A window of an East-end London church contained the inscription 'Glory to God in the highest' (Lk 2:14). But one day a little urchin threw a stone which nicked out the letter 'e', and then it read, 'Glory to God in the High st.'

Jesus got through to people on their wavelength. For some older folk we may need a 'Radio 3' wavelength and Authorized Version, while for some younger ones a 'Radio 1' approach and modern English. The message is the same, and only the Holy Spirit can open people's eyes (1 Cor 2:13–14), but the methods will vary.

Every time we launch we take one step forward. Sometimes at meetings I have encouraged people to do this. We have waited on the Lord in silence and he has shown particular steps to some, then those ministering have laid hands on them and prayed the Lord would equip each for taking that next step. As a result one lady prayed aloud for the first time in a meeting. Another, after hearing the Lord say to her, 'Feed my lambs' (Jn 21:15), offered to work with young people. Others have launched out towards full-time ministries.

It is Jesus Christ who holds the six keys to healing: faith, guidance, love, gifts, release of power and willingness to change. As we launch out we will find we need them and he will hand them to us. It's then up to us to apply them.

Now is the time to launch. Now is the time to obey Jesus' command, 'Heal the sick' (Mt 10:8). Now is the time to say, 'In the name of Jesus, be made whole!'

Suggested readings: Luke 5:1–11; 14:12–24.

Launch out into the Deep
(Lk 5:4)

Look at the open sea!
    Think of the Saviour's word!
Launch out into the deep
    And find that he's a faithful Lord.
Why do you mend your nets?
    Is it for show or gain?
Launch out into the deep
    And find that God will make it plain.

Don't look around at men!
    Think of the Saviour's power!
Launch out into the deep
    And find he's with you every hour.
Fish are not caught on land,
    Nor in the shallow sea;
Launch out into the deep
    And find that Jesus there will be.

Listen to Jesus' voice,
    Though you have nothing caught.
Launch out into the deep
    And find what God to you has brought.
Don't be afraid or doubt,
    Think on the Saviour's love.
Launch out into the deep
    And find he'll keep your head above.

Look at the other boats!
    You're not the only ones!
Launch out into the deep
    And fish together with God's sons.
Let down your nets for him,
    You'll be surprised and glad.
You will come home with such
    A catch as thrills the heart of God!

Appendix

Forty Promises of Healing from Scripture

These are each best read in their original contexts, but they have also been of great blessing and comfort to many sick and needy people as they have prayerfully claimed them in connection with their particular needs and they have been used by many Christians ministering healing in Jesus' name. Let him minister to you through them and you will know his blessing and peace. (In a few instances I have changed tenses or less colloquial phrases to allow the promises to speak directly into our hearts. These are marked AP—author's paraphrase.)

Exodus 15:26	I will not bring on you any of [these] diseases . . . for I am the Lord who heals you.
2 Kings 20:5	I have heard your prayer and seen your tears; I will heal you.
Psalm 103:3	He forgives all my sins and heals all my diseases.
Psalm 107:20	He sends out his word and heals them, and rescues them from the pit and destruction (AP).

Psalm 146:7–8   The Lord sets prisoners free, he gives sight to the blind, he straightens the backs of those that are bent.

Psalm 147:3   He heals the brokenhearted and binds up their wounds—curing their pains and their sorrows (Amplified Version).

Proverbs 3:7–8   Do not be wise in your own eyes; reverently worship the Lord and turn entirely away from evil. This will bring health to your body and nerves, and nourishment to your bones (AP).

Proverbs 4:20, 22   My son . . . listen closely to my words . . . for they are life to those who find them and health to a [person's] whole body.

Isaiah 14:24   The Lord Almighty has sworn, 'Surely, as I have planned, so it will be, and as I have purposed, so it will stand.'

Isaiah 26:3   You will keep him in perfect peace whose mind is stayed on you, because he leans on you and trusts in you (AP).

Isaiah 30:15   Thus said the Lord . . . 'In returning to Me and resting in Me you shall be saved* (healed, delivered); in quietness and in (trusting) confidence shall be your strength.' (Amplified Version.)

Isaiah 30:26   The Lord binds up the hurt of His people, and heals their wound. (Amplified Version.)

Isaiah 40:31   They that wait upon the Lord shall renew their strength; they shall mount up with wings as eagles; they shall run, and not be weary; and they shall walk, and not faint. (AV)

Isaiah 53:5 He was wounded for our transgressions, he was bruised for our iniquities; upon him was the chastisement that made us whole, and with his stripes we are healed. (RSV)

Isaiah 58:8 Then your light will break forth like the dawn, and your healing will quickly appear.

Jeremiah 17:14 Heal me, O Lord, and I shall be healed; save me, and I shall be saved; for You are my praise. (Amplified Version.)

Jeremiah 30: 13, 17 'For [the pressing together of] your wound you have no healing [device], no binding plaster . . . I will restore health to you, and I will heal your wounds,' says the Lord. (Amplified Version.)

Jeremiah 33:3, 6 Call to me and I will answer you and tell you great and unsearchable things you do not know . . . I will bring health and healing . . . I will heal my people and will let them enjoy abundant peace and security.

Ezekiel 34:16 I will search for the lost and bring back the strays. I will bind up the injured and strengthen the weak.

Matthew 6:33 Seek ye first the kingdom of God, and his righteousness; and all these things shall be added unto you. (AV)

Matthew 7:7 Keep on asking and it will be given you; keep on seeking and you will find; keep on knocking [reverently] and the door will be opened to you. (Amplified Version.)

Matthew 10:1   Jesus summoned to Him His . . . disciples and gave them power and authority over unclean spirits, to drive them out, and to cure all kinds of disease and all kinds of weakness and infirmity. (Amplified Version.)

Matthew 11:28   Come to Me, all you who . . . are . . . overburdened, and I will cause you to rest—I will ease and relieve and refresh your souls. (Amplified Version.)

Matthew 18:18–20   Whatever you bind on earth shall be bound in heaven, and whatever you loose on earth shall be loosed in heaven . . . If two of you agree on earth about anything they ask, it will be done for them by my Father in heaven. For where two or three are gathered in my name, there am I in the midst of them. (RSV)

Matthew 21:21   If you have faith and do not doubt, not only can you do what was done to the fig-tree, but also you can say to this mountain, 'Go, throw yourself into the sea,' and it will be done.

Mark 9:23   All things are possible to him [her] who believes. (RSV)

Mark 11:24   Whatever you ask for in prayer, believe that you have received it, and it will be yours.

Mark 16:17–18   These signs will accompany those who believe: In my name they will drive out demons; they will speak in new tongues . . . they will place their hands on sick people, and they will get well.

Luke 4:18–19
(cf. Isaiah 61:1–2)
The Spirit of the Lord is upon Me, because He has anointed Me to preach the good news . . . to the poor; He has sent Me to announce release to the captives, and recovery of sight to the blind; (to bind up the brokenhearted, to set the downtrodden free) those who are oppressed . . . bruised, crushed and broken down by calamity; to proclaim (that this is the day when salvation and the free favours of God are supplied in abundance) (Amplified Version, AP in brackets).

Luke 8:50
Don't be afraid; only believe, and she [he] will be well. (Good News Bible.)

John 14:12–13
Anyone who has faith in me will do what I have been doing. He will do even greater things than these, because I am going to the Father. And I will do whatever you ask in my name, so that the Son may bring glory to the Father.

Acts 2:21
Everyone who calls on the name of the Lord will be saved* [healed, delivered].

Acts 16:30–31
What must I do to be saved?* [healed, delivered] . . . Believe in the Lord Jesus, and you will be saved* [healed, delivered]—you and your household.

Ephesians 3:20
By the power at work within us [he]

is able to do far more abundantly than all that we ask or think. (RSV)

Philippians 4:6–7 Have no anxiety about anything, but in everything by prayer and supplication with thanksgiving let your requests be made known to God. And the peace of God, which passes all understanding, will keep your hearts and your minds in Christ Jesus. (RSV)

Philippians 4:13, 19 I can do all things in him who strengthens me . . . And my God will supply every need of yours according to his riches in glory in Christ Jesus. (RSV)

Hebrews 13:5–6, 8 God has said, 'Never will I leave you; never will I forsake you.' So we say with confidence, 'The Lord is my helper; I will not be afraid . . . Jesus Christ is the same yesterday and today and for ever.'

James 1:5 If you want to know what God wants you to do, ask him, and he will gladly tell you, for he is always ready to give a generous supply of wisdom to all who ask him; he will not resent it. (Living Bible.)

James 5:14–16 Is anyone sick? He should call for the church elders and they should pray over him and anoint him with oil in the name of the Lord. And the prayer of faith will save* [heal, deliver] the sick person, and the Lord will raise him [her] up. And if his [her] sickness was caused by some sin, the Lord will forgive.

Confess your faults to one another and pray for one another so that you may be healed. The earnest, fervent prayer of a person right with the Lord makes tremendous power available, is dynamic in its working, and has wonderful results (AP).

1 Peter 5:7   Cast all your anxiety on him because he cares for you.

*The same Greek word can often either be translated saved, healed or delivered, according to its context.

Index

God Wants You Whole

The Way to Healing, Health and Wholeness

by Selwyn Hughes

If God is always willing to heal, why do people remain ill—even when they have faith for healing?

How can we all live more healthy lives, day by day?

With openness and honesty, Selwyn Hughes faces squarely the issues of health and healing that concern every one of us. He examines the most common causes of ill health and the reasons we fail to receive God's healing grace. Here we see how our Creator has lovingly provided all we need for wholeness of living, if only we set ourselves to live in accordance with his will.

Above all, this book shows that even when healing eludes us and our condition is not remedied quickly, we can still rest secure in the knowledge that our heavenly Father is committed to our good—in spirit, mind, emotions, and body.

Also by Selwyn Hughes in Kingsway paperback:
A friend in Need; How to Live the Christian Life; The Christian Counsellor's Pocket Guide; Everyday Reflections; A New Heart; Marriage as God Intended.

Kingsway Publications